DEMENTIA GUIDE

Practical Ways For Caregivers To Overcome Stress During The Three Stages Of Dementia

Atwater McDaniel

Contents

Introduction   v

1. DEMENTIA, AN OVERVIEW   1
Types of Dementia   8
Who is at Risk for Alzheimer's Disease?   17

2. UNDERSTANDING THE STAGES OF DEMENTIA   23
Looking at the Early Stage   23
Knowing What to Expect from the Beginning   24
Identifying the Early Signs of Dementia   25
Considering the Middle Stage   26
Recognizing the Onset of Dementia   26
Understanding the Progression of Symptoms   26
Identifying the Late Stage   28
Knowing It's the Final Chapter   28
Moving Towards the End of Life   29

3. CHANGING THE ROLES   31
Changing Roles   32
Relationships Stressed   32
Teamwork Is Important   32
Changing Relationships   33
What Can You Do to Assist If You Are Not the Primary Caregiver?   51
Your Job and Caregiving   53
Your Children   54
Preparing and Teaching Young Children What to Expect   56

4. PROVIDING CARE DURING THE ONSET STAGE   58
The Experience of Loss   58
Overcoming Resistance   60
Discussing Diagnosis   61
Get a Second Opinion   62

Work-Related Issues   63
Lifestyle Modification   64
Relationship Issues   67

5. PROVIDING CARE THROUGH THE MIDDLE
STAGE   72
Maintaining a Schedule of Daily Activities   73
Increasing Care Needs   77
Supervision   77

6. ADVANCED STAGES OF CAREGIVING   86
Gems for Understanding Neurological Disorder   87
Supervision   90
Is therapy still required?   90
Remaining Engaged in Positive and Energizing
Activities   91
Life-Ending Problems   93
End Stage Treatment Decisions   94
Tube Feeding Pros and Cons   95
Brain Donation   96

7. THE CAREGIVER   97

8. LEGAL ISSUES   103
Decision Making   103
Durable Power of Attorney   105
Governance and Competency   106
Prior Directives   108

Final Words   113
Bibliography   115

Introduction

Your motivation for caring for a loved one with dementia is most likely a heart full of love and compassion and a desire to provide the finest care possible. While being a caregiver can be a rewarding experience, it also comes with many responsibilities and problems.

The more you understand dementia's progression, the more prepared you will be to deal with the disease's cognitive, physical, social, and emotional changes. Getting better mastery of dementia and how it impacts you and your loved one will enable you to

- Adapt to behavioral and cognitive shifts
- Develop appropriate coping methods and abilities; and
- Reduce the effects of caregiver stress, burnout, and depression on you.

You must understand that dementia is not the same as Alzheimer's disease, and Alzheimer's disease is not dementia. This is especially important for caregivers to know.

Dementia is a broad term that refers to a collection of or set of signs and symptoms that can be caused by different brain illnesses or conditions. Dementia patients have been reported to be intellectually incapable of performing daily tasks such as eating, getting dressed, working, bathing, or grooming. They may lose some or all of their problem-solving skills and competence as a result of the brain damage. They may experience minor personality changes, a loss of emotional control, amnesia, memory loss, and tension or anxiety because they no longer recognize their surroundings.

On the other hand, Alzheimer's disease is just one of the disorders that can cause dementia. It is a progressive disease characterized by signs and symptoms that impact a person's memory, thinking, and behavior. Another way to explain this is: Alzheimer's disease is a cause, and dementia is a result. Alzheimer's disease isn't the only cause of dementia, it's just the most frequent.

The numerous myths and fallacies surrounding dementia and Alzheimer's disease can create issues for caregivers when caring for patients with these disorders. These opinions impact how patients are perceived, which can result in misconceptions and assumptions that may not be beneficial to the patient, and may even be harmful.

According to studies, 24 million people are living with dementia. Understanding dementia and the stages of this illness will help you to make informed decisions about dementia care. Many people are unaware that there are over 100 different varieties of dementia, even though dementia is one of the world's fastest-increasing diseases. As stated, Alzheimer's disease is the most frequent type of memory loss disease among those over the age of 65. In the United States, dementia is the sixth largest cause of mortality. The figures are grim, given its enormous aging population. It is estimated that 10 million Baby Boomers will develop dementia at some point in their lives.

As the world's life expectancy continues to rise, we are increasingly confronted with new difficulties that we must address as a society. Consider this: the prevalence of health issues such as dementia and its associated illnesses rises as people age. These illnesses present numerous obstacles not only to the patient but also to the patient's family and the caretakers of the afflicted.

Furthermore, statistics show that women live longer than males; as a result, science predicts one in every twenty women over the age of 65 and one in every five women over the age of 80 will develop dementia. According to studies, 70% of persons diagnosed with dementia live at home and are cared for by family and friends. The figures for family caregivers/care partners are similarly alarming. Half of all family caregivers/care partners get major illnesses, and some caregivers die before the dementia patient, leaving them behind with no one to care for them.

Understanding the signs of dementia, the many dementia types, and the various dementia phases is required to successfully provide care at home for a person with a diagnosis of dementia. Agitation, hostility, and wrath, for example, are behaviors that many people with dementia or age-related memory loss disease would exhibit to some degree. A little-known fact that many people are unaware of is that some people have more than one type of dementia. This is a common occurrence, and in fact, Alzheimer's disease and vascular dementia can coexist in the same person.

What should you do if someone's memory appears to be fading over time? How do you look after a loved one who is losing his or her ability to communicate effectively and function independently due to a loss of information processing ability? If you've ever lived with someone who has dementia, you'll understand how emotionally, physically, and cognitively draining it can be. All of this asserts a lot of stress and pressure on caregivers and their families, making it nearly impossible to live a happy and fulfilled life. Dementia causes enormous changes in the family structure, which are often marked by a sequence of losses, making any attempts to adjust too difficult to bear.

However, as you are well aware, one of the first steps in winning any fight is to understand your adversary. As a caregiver, having a good understanding of what life with dementia entails may be the biggest sigh of relief you'll ever breathe. With that, you'll be well-prepared to offer assistance to such patients, or, better yet, you'll have some coping strategies for navigating through such tumultuous times.

The numerous myths and fallacies surrounding dementia and Alzheimer's disease result in misinformation for the caregivers of dementia patients. These myths impact how patients are perceived, and create misconceptions and assumptions that may not be beneficial to the patient, or may even be harmful.

Caring is a caregiver's fundamental responsibility; it is the foundation of the entire profession. Caring does not solely imply passively supplying what is physically required, nor does it include simply doing what is asked of you. Caring is about creating ties and a sense of kinship with healthcare professionals, caretakers, and clients on a deeper level. These partnerships serve as conduits for therapeutic care that holistically benefits all the people involved.

The ability to empathize is the one quality that genuinely distinguishes a caretaker. If you are in this situation, as you provide care, consider how you would like to be treated and try to put yourself in the metaphorical shoes of a dementia patient. Doing so will help you to provide empathetic, compassionate and appropriate care.

For a dedicated caregiver to accomplish all of this, it is necessary to remove any preconceived views about Alzheimer's disease and dementia that have developed because of public misconceptions. It is important that you educate yourself. Know the facts and truths about every idea of care: who you're caring for, what to expect, how to treat them, and the importance of long-term care. My hope is that by reading this, you will not only gain important information but also gain confidence in your ability to provide the best possible treatment. With this knowledge, you will be able to take control, manage the symptoms of this disease as they arise, and cope effectively with the continuing changes. Above all, recognize that you are not alone; many other individuals are going through the same things you are.

I've provided information on each type of dementia because there are so many distinct types of dementia and stages of dementia. This can help you better understand how to give your family member the best possible care and how to ask the proper questions about future care needs. This knowledge will also equip you to act as an advocate for someone who is suffering from dementia. Dementia manifests itself in different ways in different people. This will have an impact on how you approach and deliver care.

So, let's get started on your dementia education adventure. I hope you will discover things in this book that are not only informative but which also give you the confidence that you are providing the greatest care possible.

Chapter 1

Dementia, An Overview

As we discussed in the introduction, dementia is not the name of a specific disease. Dementia is a catch-all term for a collection of symptoms, most of which are cognitive. The word itself does not uniquely identify any specific disease, just as the word *automobile* does not describe individual brands or models, and *vegetable* does not describe just one of the items in a salad bar. So *dementia* enumerates the many and varied symptoms that might be seen in the condition of an afflicted person.

Alzheimer's disease is the most occurring form of dementia, followed by vascular dementia, mixed dementia (both Alzheimer's and vascular), Lewy Body dementia, Frontotemporal dementia, Parkinson's Disease dementia, and others. There are more than 50 dementia diseases in all, according to some sources. We'll discuss them in more detail below.

Before we do, it's important to understand that dementia is a chronic condition that worsens with time. This means that the chemistry and structure of brain neurons, as well as the connections between them, continue to deteriorate until the individual passes. It is sometimes referred to as *brain failure*, just like heart failure, kidney failure, or other organ failures. The ability to think, including the ability to remember, communicate, reason, and understand, progressively decline.

Dementia is a term used to explain a deterioration in memory function that is severe enough to interfere with daily life. Currently, dementia has no cure and nothing can be done to slow its progression. Sadly, the life expectancy of the loved one who is affected will be shortened. It's encouraging to realize that effective caregiving can greatly reduce the severity of symptoms and the well-being of your loved one with dementia.

Although no two persons with dementia progress in the same way, most go through the same three stages: mild, moderate, and severe dementia. The best way to deal with each stage is to be prepared and armed with coping techniques by understanding the evolution and symptoms of each stage.

Signs And Symptoms:

The sufferer is usually the first to detect the signs of dementia, who often mistake it for memory loss that comes with age. The severity of symptoms will vary from person to person, and the presence of the disease and the rate at which it develops will also be unique to that individual.

Memory:

Being forgetful is expected; we forget people's names, locations we've visited, and even need to think about what we had for lunch today. However, with dementia, the forgetfulness or memory lapses do not remain as rare as in normal persons but rather increase over time. The following are signs of an dementia impairment:

- Questions and comments are repeated within a brief period after one another. Being utterly oblivious of what you've just said or that you've just posted a question and received a response.

- An inability to recall whole conversations. Missing essential events or appointments due to a lack of awareness of the date. Alternatively, attending these appointments and events but forgetting about them later.
- Constantly misplacing items. Putting something in an unusual spot and then trying to find it because there's no memory of where it was placed. This holds true for even the most common of objects, such as a watch, a pair of glasses or a cane.
- Forgetting the names of common things and having difficulty recognizing and naming family members.

Disorientation:

With dementia, memory lapses combined with an impaired sense of surroundings can often lead to disorientation. For example, a patient may be completely unaware of the time, which can affect sleeping patterns; they may be unaware of the day and dress inappropriately for an occasion they believe is occurring. or they may be unaware of the season, which can cause a patient to dress inappropriately for summer or winter thinking it is either one. Disorientation can cause a patient to feel lost even in the most familiar of environments, such as their home or their place of care.

Using Phrases:

A person with dementia may find it difficult to talk and express themselves with the few words they still have due to a loss of understanding of common object names and the forgetting of basic vocabulary. Of course, results in the eventual loss of writing skills as letter strokes are forgotten, and the ability to hold a pen or pencil properly, and other fine motor skills eventually decline.

Keeping a Record:

Keeping track of and thinking about common daily responsibilities like paying bills, feeding pets, catering to personal hygiene, watering the flowers, and so on is also a cause of dementia, where a person's impaired memory creates gaps in their train of thought that cannot be filled because the sufferer would not know what it was or what had to be done in the first place.

Judgment:

For a person with dementia, an impeded mode of judgment for ordinary everyday decisions like where to park, what brand to buy at the grocery store, and so on can be quite stressful. This lack of adequate judgment can put a person into a scenario in which he could be injured.

Planning:

When planning is disrupted, everything that requires steps is disrupted, such as getting dressed, where the first step is to put your head through the shirt, then each arm, and finally pull it down. Cooking processes, to-do lists, what to buy, and anything else that requires steps become hampered, and patients become upset, confused, and frustrated with the fact that they are doing things wrong that are normal and intended to be straightforward and routine become hampered.

Changes in Personality:

Dementia affects not only a person's daily routines and thinking methods but also how they feel. And emotions, in any form, can lead to long-term issues such as:

- Reluctance to interact with others
- Suffering from depression
- Mood fluctuations caused by bipolar disorder
- Getting agitated easily
- Having wrath or agitation outbursts
- Sleep disturbances/ sleep deprivation
- Getting lost during conversation and going off on a tangent
- Losing inhibitions

- Experiencing hallucinations
- People and events that cause irrational distress

Knowing the signs of dementia will help you detect whether what a patient is feeling or going through is due to the disease or his own personality and agitation as a caregiver. Knowing and understanding these signs and symptoms might be the difference between recognizing the presence of a disease and its consequences and assuming that a person is merely anxious, irritable, or unpleasant. Recognizing the presence of an illness through the behavior of patients is the first step toward comprehending them.

Many of the signs and symptoms of dementia are similar to those of other medical conditions.

Dementia symptoms like mental confusion, forgetfulness, or memory issues may result from another medical illness in an elderly person. Dementia is not the only diagnosis that may be made based on these symptoms. It will be easier to distinguish between dementia and other forms of memory loss if you are aware of these medical illnesses and their symptoms. These illnesses include:

- **Infection Of the urinary tract**

When a senior adult exhibits indicators of heightened moodiness and unexpected mental confusion, the first thing that comes to mind is that they require a urinalysis to rule out a UTI. Infections can be treated, and the disorientation and memory issues that an aging senior may have can be reversed. When a family member of an elderly senior notices an increase in perplexity, it is usual practice for a doctor to request a urinalysis. Irritability and mental disorientation will be reduced if the infection is properly treated.

- ## **Lack of proper nutrition or malnutrition**

It's crucial to check into your family member's refrigerators frequently when you visit them at home. Look for expired products and food that has gone bad. Examine the cabinets to see what they're eating or preparing for themselves. The importance of a proper diet for the body and brain function cannot be overstated. Memory loss, disorientation, sluggishness, and a sense of apathy in everyday tasks might be caused by decreased food intake or an inadequate intake of vitamins and minerals. Some people even have Meals on Wheels delivered but don't consume the entire meal because they share it with their pets. So that this does not happen, ensure the pet has food.

- ## **Lack of sleep or sleep deprivation**

Our body and mind work differently when we don't get enough sleep. The importance of a good night's sleep for our physical and mental health cannot be overstated. Sleep and waking cycles will be disrupted in those who are showing signs and symptoms of dementia. Establishing a sleep schedule is critical to promote sleep and reduce the consequences of sleep deprivation. It's also critical for the caregiver of a dementia patient to obtain enough sleep and rest.

- ## **Liver disease**

Our liver is in charge of purifying our blood. It converts the compounds we ingest in the form of food and medication into a non-toxic form that may be absorbed into the bloodstream. The liver loses its ability to filter poisons as it becomes inefficient. Toxin levels in the body will build with time, affecting all body organs, including brain function. The mental bewilderment that results is irrevocable.

- **Low Blood Sugar or Hypoglycemia**

Hypoglycemia, often known as low blood sugar, can make a person irritable. When a person's blood sugar dips because they haven't eaten, personality changes and short-term mental disorientation might ensue. These signs and symptoms may appear to be dementia symptoms, but they aren't. Restoring blood sugar levels to normal by having a person drink juice or eat a peanut butter sandwich to alleviate the symptoms.

- **Low Thyroid Levels or Under-Active Thyroid**

Low thyroid levels are likely to be disregarded when doctors are trying to figure out what's causing memory loss. The thyroid gland produces a lot of hormones that control human body temperature, metabolism, and other processes. Hypothyroidism, or low thyroid levels, can cause symptoms such as memory loss, depression, hair loss, dry skin, weight gain, constipation, and irritability. When treated with medication, these symptoms can be reversed.

- **Medications**

All aging elders need to be aware of their medications and how to keep them safe. Many drugs can produce disorientation or short-term memory loss, and some drugs prescribed for the elderly have the opposite effect. The majority of drug-induced bouts of confusion can be rectified by stopping the medicine, having the prescribing doctor modify the dosage, or continuing to take it as prescribed.

- **Seizures**

When the brain's electrical conduction or communication becomes disordered and overstimulated, seizures occur. People who have frequent and severe seizures are more likely to acquire dementia. When a person stops breathing during a seizure, this becomes more likely. Brain injury may be irreversible if there is a lack of oxygen to the brain. It's crucial to remember that those who have been diagnosed with dementia have a higher chance of having seizures as the condition develops.

- **Substance abuse, long-term drug addiction**

Misuse of illegal substances or prescription prescriptions, like alcohol abuse, disrupts normal brain function. Drugs disrupt brain function and cause the death of brain cells. Individuals who have struggled with substance misuse for a long time are at significant risk of acquiring dementia. This condition can be reversed if the abuse is stopped before serious damage occurs.

Types of Dementia

Dementia is caused by a variety of disorders that induce brain dysfunction. Each disease has its way of causing brain cell death, and each has its pattern, such as where it starts in the brain and which parts of the brain it impacts the most. Diseases differ in their effects on people's rate of decline as they progress.

You'll find descriptions of the primary disorders that cause dementia in this section, and their ranking shows how common they are in the United States. We'll start with the most prevalent dementias, then move on to less frequent types.

Being fair to yourself in this circumstance entails not trying to process all of these diseases and information at once. The last thing you can do is to be concerned about every variety of dementia and if you're dealing with one of them. It's wise to leave the armchair diagnosis to football fans.

ALZHEIMER'S DISEASE

Alzheimer's disease (AD) is the most prevalent cause of dementia, affecting 60 to 80 percent of those who have the disease. The condition is caused by specific proteins developing in the brain known as *amyloid* and *tau*.

Plaques and tangles arise due to these aberrant amyloid and tau deposits. Amyloid plaques resemble blobs, and tau tangles resemble protein threads. Both forms cause brain cells to stop working correctly, resulting in dementia.

Memory loss is a common sign of Alzheimer's disease, which is thought to begin in the hippocampus, the brain region that controls most memory. Other signs of Alzheimer's disease include difficulty finding words, impatience, and confusion.

With millions of people living with AD and millions more on the verge of developing it, the race is on to decipher how AD begins and how to stop it. This problem has eluded an answer for a long time because the human brain contains more cells than stars in the galaxy.

There are currently just a few medical treatment options. These methods do not cure; nevertheless, they may help halt the disease's progression. AD, like most dementia-causing brain disorders, is currently incurable.

The most common treatment method is to begin with Donepezil (Aricept). After a few months, the doctor will add Memantine (Namenda). It isn't easy to know which drug is causing any side effects if both are begun at the same time. The most prevalent adverse effects are stomach or intestinal issues.

Despite research efforts, no new medicinal treatments for Alzheimer's disease have been developed since 2003. This fact alone demonstrates how difficult it is to discover a remedy, and prevention is our best hope till something changes.

The same precautions we take for heart health should be taken for brain health. Controlling high blood pressure, maintaining a healthy weight, and exercising frequently are all examples of these methods.

People with Alzheimer's disease usually survive from 3 to 11 years after being diagnosed. However, that's a generalization; some people do not live even that long after being diagnosed, while others live for up to 20 years. We never know the amount of time we have left when we have cognitive failure due to dementia.

VASCULAR DEMENTIA

The mechanism of vascular dementia differs from that of other types of dementia. Vascular dementia is not a disease that progresses over time. It is caused by alterations in the blood vessels that feed the brain, which reduce blood flow to brain cells. Brain cells are obnoxious little scavengers, and cells die quickly when their supply of oxygen and other vital components is interrupted.

When there are blockages in the vessels caused by plaque or breaks, blood flow to the brain slows or stops. A stroke can occur if the halt in flow lasts for a long time or is extensive. Cell death that isn't caused by a full-blown stroke, on the other hand, is significantly more common and can lead to dementia.

A blood flow restriction may be only brief. The plaque obstructing blood flow can detach from the blood vessel wall and float to a larger blood vessel, allowing blood flow to resume. This event is responsible for some of a person's day-to-day fluctuations in dementia symptoms. Mini-strokes, also known as transient ischemic events, are caused by brief blockages.

Blood leaks into the tissues when blood vessels in the brain leak or tear. The brain is crammed into a small space inside the skull, and the brain has nowhere to go as the blood accumulation increases. Inside the brain, pressure rises, impairing or killing cells. When enough cells in the brain die or malfunction, dementia develops.

Vascular dementia can be caused by any chronic health condition that damages blood vessels. Uncontrolled diabetes and hypertension are the worst culprits. Controlling these factors is crucial in preventing or treating vascular dementia. Doctors may prescribe blood thinners to select patients to prevent clots in the brain.

Vascular dementia can manifest itself in any part of the brain. As a result, the symptoms differ based on the affected area. The course of vascular dementia is challenging to predict because of these variances in location.

LEWY BODY DEMENTIA

Another kind of dementia is Lewy body dementia (LBD). A Lewy body is a protein clump known as *alpha-synuclein*. For unexplained reasons, Lewy bodies form, and their impact is determined by where they originate in the brain.

The most common symptom of LBD is difficulty moving. Muscle stiffness, tremors, and a shuffling gait are all common symptoms. Parkinson's disease is likely to be diagnosed in the affected person. More unusual symptoms emerge with time, ruling out a primary Parkinson's diagnosis.

The symptoms of LBD are distinct from those of other dementias. Visual hallucinations, sleep disturbances, and difficulties doing mental tasks are among them. The memory is usually unaffected.

Sleep problems are common in people with LBD. REM sleep disorder creates strange sleep patterns that appear to be a person acting out their dreams. They may talk in their sleep, have violent movements, or fall out of bed. Symptoms of sleep deprivation sometimes appear years before other symptoms develop.

The autonomic nervous system is frequently affected by dementia with Lewy bodies. Blood pressure, heart rate, perspiration, and digestion are all controlled by this system. Dizziness and gastrointestinal problems, such as recurrent constipation, are dysfunction symptoms.

When a person's blood pressure drops due to LBD they may have a brief blackout, which can lead to falls. The person has no recollection of the cause of the fall due to the blackout.

There are no treatments to reverse or slow LBD, as there are for most kinds of dementia. The objective of medical treatment is to control symptoms, yet some drugs have the opposite effect. Because of this, a lot of people with the condition are unable to take a wide range of drugs.

The use of LBD anti-drugs for Parkinson's frequently results in a worsening of behavioral symptoms. Antipsychotic medicines, which are supposed to calm you down, can make you more agitated and aggressive. Any drug given to someone with LBD should be carefully chosen and monitored.

It's hard to say how long someone with LBD will live. The average time between diagnosis and death is 2 to 12 years. The faster the disease progresses, the younger the person is at diagnosis. In addition, it tends to progress faster in women than in men.

MIXED DEMENTIA

A person with mixed dementia has more than one of the dementia-causing brain diseases. In mixed dementia, the most common combination is VD and AD, and this combination is found in most dementia patients over the age of 80. It's difficult to tell how much each disease contributes to a person's symptoms when they have mixed dementia. The general standard of care for each disease is medical treatment.

FRONTOTEMPORAL DEMENTIA

When the frontal and temporal lobes of the brain shrink due to cell damage caused by the protein tau or another protein called TDP-43, frontotemporal dementia (FTD) develops. The frontal and temporal lobes may have a unique affinity for these proteins.

FTD, or Pick's disease as initially known, is caused by their accumulation in specific areas.

The symptoms indicate that the frontal and temporal lobes are both dysfunctional. These lobes control the executive function—what we use to make plans, solve problems, and make decisions. The ability to do these things deteriorates as FTD progresses, and mood management, emotional control, and inhibition are all affected.

Memory problems are uncommon in FTD, but behavioral symptoms are common. Mood swings are standard, as is a complete lack of empathy. A lack of empathy can particularly hurt others, and this change can be devastating to someone who was previously loving and supportive.

Disinhibition can lead to strange behaviors and salty language out of character for a person's life. Disturbances in sleep can finally become a deal-breaker for staying at home, and Caregivers cannot function with little to no sleep for an extended period. Some people may threaten physical violence due to outbursts of rage and distrust, and this risk can serve as an additional incentive to seek full-time care.

For the underlying brain condition that causes FTD, no treatments are beneficial. Although memantine (Namenda) has helped a small number of people with FTD, studies show that it is ineffective most of the time. The main objective of treatment is to alleviate the distressing symptoms that FTD causes.

PARKINSON'S DISEASE DEMENTIA

Parkinson's disease is a neurological disorder that attacks people. The twin of dementia with Lewy bodies is dementia. Both disorders are caused by the presence of Lewy bodies in brain cells, and their symptoms are similar. Whether Parkinson's dementia and LBD are two different diseases is a point of contention among experts.

The history of Parkinson's disease is used to diagnose Parkinson's dementia. Parkinson's dementia is defined as dementia that appears at least one year following the diagnosis of Parkinson's disease. Within the first year of Parkinson's-like symptoms, LBD develops.

Unusual physical symptoms, such as visual hallucinations, yelling or thrashing while sleeping, and loss of facial expressions, occur with Parkinson's disease dementia and LBD. Drugs that would help with other dementias often worsen symptoms, and both types of dementia are treated in the same way.

CREUTZFELDT-JAKOB DISEASE

Creutzfeldt-Jakob disease (CJD) is a dementia-causing brain illness. About 350 instances are reported each year in the United States, according to the National Institutes of Health.

The vast majority of cases have an unknown cause. This type of CJD is known as sporadic CJD. A rare genetic mutation that can be passed down from parent to child affects ten to fifteen percent of those affected. Anyone with a genetic form of CJD should seek genetic counseling to learn more about the risks.

Contamination from infectious sources is the most common cause of CJD, accounting for one in every million cases. In the public's mind, CJD is linked to mad cow disease, since tainted beef has been a source of infection.

Its rapid progression characterizes CJD. From the moment of diagnosis, the average life expectancy is one year. There is no way to stop it, and symptom control and comfort care are the main goals of medical treatment.

NORMAL-PRESSURE HYDROCEPHALUS

Excess fluid buildup in the brain causes normal pressure hydrocephalus (NPH). Infections or tumors are rarely the cause of this buildup. Most of the time, there is no discernible cause. People in their 60's and 70's are more likely to develop NPH.

NPH's excess fluid pushes on surrounding brain tissues, causing mechanical damage and dementia. Mild cognitive symptoms may be misdiagnosed as other disorders. NPH also causes difficulty walking and a loss of bladder control.

If a person with NPH can endure surgery, a shunt can be implanted in the brain. A shunt is a tiny tube that connects the brain and the belly, allowing fluid to drain from the brain's small, constrained region to the immense pool of abdominal fluid.

According to studies, shunt implantation frequently corrects walking problems. After surgery, cognitive impairment and bladder control loss are common, although shunt installation may prevent further decline. Shunt placement is a routine surgery that carries some risks but is generally considered safe.

HUNTINGTON'S DISEASE

Huntington's disease (HD) is a rare form of dementia caused by a genetic mutation in the brain. The accountable gene can be passed down from one generation to the next. If a person carries the gene for HD, they will get the disease. Symptoms usually appear in the thirties or forties for those who are affected.

Severe mobility disturbances, dementia, and psychiatric illnesses are the three types of increasing HD symptoms.

HD causes significant mobility and behavioral issues, necessitating expert care 24 hours a day, seven days a week. From diagnosis, patients can expect to live for 10 to 30 years.

When a person carries the HD gene, genetic counseling can aid in family planning. A child's chances of getting the gene from an afflicted parent are 50/50. If a child does not inherit the gene, it is unlikely that their descendants will develop HD.

WERNICKE-KORSAKOFF SYNDROME

A thiamine deficiency causes Wernicke-Korsakoff syndrome (WKS). Thiamine, further referred to as vitamin B1, is a critical nutrient for brain function. Malnutrition, eating disorders, and chemotherapy can all cause thiamine shortage. The most prevalent cause is drinking, however, it can also be caused by stomach surgery, cancer, or overall malnutrition.

Thiamine insufficiency causes irreparable damage to brain cells if not treated early, and the process is not reversed by restoring vitamin levels. Mental confusion, eyesight impairments, and a lack of motor coordination are all symptoms of WKS.

WKS is characterized by disorientation, memory impairment, and the inability to form new memories. The disease has no known cure, and medical treatment can only aid with symptom management.

The diagnosis of WKS caused by drinking is challenging for families, and years of alcohol misuse are likely to have wreaked havoc on the family. When it comes to coping with WKS, the stigma associated with drinking persists.

POSTERIOR CORTICAL ATROPHY

PCA (posterior cortical atrophy) is an uncommon form of Alzheimer's disease. Its visual and spatial effects are the most prominent. The brain's posterior cortex interprets visual input. The eyes may take in images without difficulty with PCA, but the brain does not process them correctly.

The majority of PCA sufferers blame their condition on poor vision, and they seek ophthalmology treatment. However, no change in eyeglass prescription will fix the brain's inability to interpret what it sees.

PCA is characterized by difficulties reading and judging distances. It's possible that a person won't be able to tell whether an object is moving or stationary. It may be challenging to tell whether one or more objects are visible. PCA causes hallucinations in certain people.

For people between the ages of 50 and 65, PCA symptoms are most common. The disease is frequently misdiagnosed and mislabeled as Alzheimer's disease. No treatment can stop PCA from progressing.

Who is at Risk for Alzheimer's Disease?

Though Alzheimer's disease is more frequently associated with the old, it is not age-related and can affect anyone at risk of developing it. Here you will learn more about the different types of people who may or may not develop Alzheimer's disease.

Age:

It has been established that adults over 65 are more likely to get Alzheimer's disease. By the age of 85, half of the elderly population will have Alzheimer's disease. Early indications and symptoms of Alzheimer's disease can appear in someone's 40s or 50s.

Genetics:

It has been proved through genetic tests that having a family with Alzheimer's increases your chances of obtaining the condition yourself. The danger increases the closer the relative is to you, such as a parent. Studies on genes have shown a unique mutation that, when present, ensures a person's genetically transferred Alzheimer's disease, even if they are not aware of it at the time.

Gender:

According to statistics, women are more likely than males to get Alzheimer's disease. However, you must consider that women are statistically proven to live longer than men and so have a more considerable risk of Alzheimer's disease.

Mild Cognitive Impairment:

Mild Cognitive Impairment, or MCI, refers to a state in which persons have an abnormally high amount of memory loss for their age. Alzheimer's disease and dementia are more common in persons with MCI. Healthy living through exercise, a balanced diet, adequate rest, and suitable medication precautions should be performed and done by anyone with MCI to avoid the onset of Alzheimer's or Dementia.

Head Trauma:

Anything that affects the brain or the head area can cause problems with the brain's functioning. Trauma to the head, such as being in a car accident, can cause Alzheimer's disease.

Lifestyle:

When it comes to any sickness, one of the contributing factors to any unfortunate events is always lifestyle. There have been no established correlations between lifestyle and the onset of Alzheimer's disease. However, because there have been established correlations between heart disease and Alzheimer's disease, we can deduce that the lifestyle choices that cause heart disease are also one of the suspected causes of Alzheimer's disease. The following will be included:

- Not getting enough exercise
- Smoking
- Hypertension - state where the blood pressure is abnormally high.
- High cholesterol levels in the blood
- Diabetes that is untreated or poorly treated
- Eating habits that are harmful to one's health
- Distancing oneself from others socially.

Diagnosis:

Diagnosing Alzheimer's disease has no definite and sure-fire method, just like everything related to Alzheimer's, such as its cause and cure. A doctor will identify a patient with this disease based on his observations, the patient's or relative's remarks about what they've noticed, and some more medical testing. Only after death, when brain matter is examined under a microscope for plaque and tangles, can the presence of Alzheimer's disease be determined.

Physical Examinations:

The physical tests that a doctor will do on you will be designed to assess your neurological condition. This is what these workouts will be about.

- Reflexes
- Muscle vigor
- Hearing and vision
- Balance or equilibrium
- Good eye-hand coordination
- Being able to stand up and walk in a straight line on your own.

Lab tests:

Memory lapses can be caused by a variety of factors other than Alzheimer's disease, such as thyroid or vitamin shortages. It is not rare for a doctor to conduct lab tests not just for Alzheimer's disease but for anything else in order to rule out other prospective medical issues as well as existing issues that may contribute to the presence of Alzheimer's disease or its impact on the patient's overall health.

Mental Exam:

This isn't the kind of mental test you'd have to sit through before a job interview. When Alzheimer's disease is suspected, a mental exam takes around 10 minutes and assesses a person's memory and thinking patterns.

Neuropsychological Exam:

If your doctor thinks it's necessary, a neuropsychological examination will take second place to a mental examination. This is a longer version of the mental exam that may take several hours to complete. Its objective is to examine your mental abilities to recall information and your thought process. When the findings are available, they will be compared to those of other persons your age. This test can assist diagnose dementia in its early stages, allowing for better preparation for the mid- and later phases. This evaluation can also predict the types of dementia a person may have, allowing for the required preparations, such as activities and medication options, to be made ahead of time.

Imaging of the Brain:

The purpose of brain imaging is to detect any anomalies in the brain's size or function. This method is also utilized to detect any pre-existing brain injuries, such as strokes, tumors, or previous trauma. The following types of brain imaging will be used:

- CT Scan — A Computerized Tomography scan examines your brain in slices or cross-sections to look for abnormalities. The patient will be instructed to lie flat and remain still on a tiny panel that will slide into the CT scan machine throughout this procedure. After you've settled in, X-rays will be used to scan your brain.

- MRI – magnetic resonance imaging is routinely used in the Alzheimer's diagnosis procedure to rule out other factors that could be causing memory lapses or altering brain function. MRI testing, unlike CT scanning, uses radio waves to make images of your brain that physicians believe can help them diagnose Alzheimer's disease in the future by detecting any shrinkage.

- PET – positron emission tomography (PET) uses a very
  low-level radioactive tracer (which will not hurt you) to
  see through the scan where the blood flow is going
  through your brain. Doctors can use a PET scan to see if
  your brain is functioning normally and to check for
  plaque, which is one of the most common causes of
  Alzheimer's.

Future Tests:

Studies are continually being undertaken in the field of
Alzheimer's disease on all facets of the disease. One of these
studies is focused on testing and the development of potentially
better testing methods for determining the risk of Alzheimer's
disease. These are some of the possibilities:

- Advancements in brain imaging - to capture brain
  shrinkage in its exact proportions rather than merely a
  picture of the brain.
- More incompetent mental exams - mental exams to
  better detect Alzheimer's disease. Doctors are conducting
  a study to determine what to include and question a
  person to arrive at an Alzheimer's diagnosis.
- The use of biomarkers to identify whether or not plaque
  is present or has the potential to form by measuring
  protein levels in the blood or spinal fluid.

If you or a loved one has been diagnosed with Alzheimer's disease,
keep in mind that not all of these tests will be performed;
nonetheless, the testing procedure will almost certainly
incorporate one or more of the above-mentioned approaches.

*A few months after retirement, my mother moved in with us for a while. Since
she was living alone and had nothing to do at the moment, she was a woman
of few words and razor-sharp wit. One day I realized that she would say or
ask the same thing more than one. She also started losing her cool over minor
issues; I was beginning to feel worried and felt something was off. One day she*

was walking to the grocery store in the nearby town, and she completely forgot where she was going and was found walking alone on the highway and was brought home by the police. In a different scenario, she would often forget what day it was or even the time of the day, and when asked, she would dismiss me, saying "I'm getting old, who needs to keep track of these things," and when I suggested we see a doctor she would hear none of it.

One day she was looking for her phone in the house and all this time she was looking for it. She was busy talking to someone on it. This was when she realized she was having a "senior moment "and became more concerned with her memory. She finally agreed to see the doctor when she again thought she had lost the house keys, and she had them in her hands while turning her bag upside down.

Chapter 2

Understanding The Stages Of Dementia

Dementia is a progressive disease in all its forms. And while this decrease is frequently viewed as a continual process rather than a one-time event, it is, in fact, a one-time event.

To better understand how symptoms evolve during the disease, it's helpful to divide it into early, middle, and late stages.

The lines between these stages are, predictably, blurred, and each person experiences dementia differently, depending on his personality before illness, any other medical illnesses he may have, and whether he receives adequate assistance. However, the stages I've described are still a solid general guide to what to expect in the months and years after a diagnosis.

I begin by discussing dementia in general, using Alzheimer's disease as an example, and then move on to vascular dementia, frontotemporal dementia, and Lewy body disease for more precise details.

Looking at the Early Stage

Because it encompasses some of the very first symptoms that a person may exhibit when he develops dementia, this stage has unusually hazy borders. These could be new symptoms that emerge out of nowhere or a progression of a mild cognitive impairment that has been present for some time. In either case, symptoms will likely appear in a different order and at a different pace in different people. Nonetheless, the following parts detail the behaviors and symptoms to be aware of. Everyone is unique, and dementia manifests itself in different ways in each of us.

Knowing What to Expect from the Beginning

It would be so much easier for doctors, patients, and their families if diseases always followed their textbook descriptions to the letter. In that manner, diagnosing any medical ailment would be a breeze, therapy could begin sooner, and patients would be in better shape. But, in illness and health, life isn't like that. Early dementia is no exception.

People can present with a wide range of early symptoms. Some persons exhibit symptoms that perplex their doctors at first, and they remain medical mysteries for a while before a diagnosis is made (often because their symptoms could easily be due to a host of other conditions). Others, meanwhile, show up at their doctor's office with the diagnosis seemingly tattooed on their foreheads because it's so obvious to see.

Early dementia has two fundamental effects on someone, regardless of how it manifests: *change* and *loss*. Memory, mood, demeanor, and capacity to manage day-to-day living will all show signs of deterioration. Not only does a person with early-stage dementia physically lose belongings and memories, but you may also realize that you're losing some of your relationship with him, as well as him losing aspects of what made him who he is.

It's a good idea to prepare for the unexpected because you never know how dementia will manifest itself.

Identifying the Early Signs of Dementia

Memory loss is the most common reason for patients to go to the doctor, or to be escorted to the doctor. The most common problem is forgetting names, faces, dates, appointments, directions to known places, and specifics of recent events.

People frequently note that their relative, friend, or spouse is having difficulty following the thread of conversation when conversing with him, and/or that he keeps saying the same things over and over, as if for the first time, or repeating the same questions.

Difficulty managing change: Any break from one's typical routine, as well as the adoption of new ideas, can be difficult to deal with. This shift is especially obvious in persons who have always been willing to take on new challenges or adaptive in terms of experimenting with various methods. Likewise, people who are trapped in their ways can get even more stuck. Another early indicator could be procrastination in making decisions such as where to go on vacation and what to buy when out shopping, what to order from a restaurant menu, and what clothes to wear to work or out for the evening.

In early dementia, losing things can become the norm rather than the exception, and might involve misplacing objects such as keys, reading glasses, and television remote controls regularly.

Poor judgment: Simple monetary transactions can be perplexing, and persons with early dementia are more prone to fall for a bargain or sign up for an insurance policy or mobile phone contract that they don't require.

Low mood, anxiety, uncertainty, mood swings, impatience, and a withdrawal from regular social activities can all be early dementia signs.

Considering the Middle Stage

Please accept my apologies for seeming redundant about dementia's unpredictability, but the time between the onset of the early stages and progression into the intermediate stages can vary greatly. Obviously, it would be. It would be much more orderly if each stage lasted a set number of years, allowing sufferers and their caregivers to plan ahead with some precision. But dementia isn't so forgiving, and while some people can linger in the early stages for years, others can speed through it and notice a rapid deterioration in their symptoms.

Recognizing the Onset of Dementia

The symptoms that arrived and fluctuate randomly in the first stage become more permanent in the middle stage, and their onset accelerates. As a result, persons in this stage frequently experience memory problems, struggle with daily tasks like cooking, shopping, and dressing, and show much more noticeable shifts in their mood and behavior.

It becomes increasingly clear that these shifts aren't due to senior moments or the assumed inevitability of a decline into eccentricity and increased grumpiness as one gets older. It's evident that something is wrong at this point, and medical guidance on what's going on and what can rightfully be done about it is now required.

Understanding the Progression of Symptoms

The symptoms that were present in the first stage are now more severe, and the following scenarios are more likely:

- **Memory loss:** As this symptom worsens, sufferers frequently forget the names of family members and friends, miss appointments, and put themselves and others in danger by, for example, leaving pots cooking on

the stove, eating expired food, or leaving the front door
open.

- **Conversational issues:** Repetition can become the
  norm in conversations, or people with dementia in the
  later stages may not bother to participate since they can't
  understand what's being said. They may also struggle to
  find the correct words for items and instead describe
  them; for example, a watch becomes 'the time-telling
  thing on my arm.' Confabulation - filling in memory gaps
  with erroneous details that they perceive to be genuine –
  is also common at this stage. When asked what happened
  the previous night, for example, they give a version of
  events that bears little reference to reality but is
  convincing nonetheless.

- **Losing stuff:** The most typical objects to go missing in
  the middle stages of dementia are the dementia sufferers
  themselves. Wandering is widespread, and it often results
  in people being unable to locate their intended
  destination or return home. It's not uncommon to lose
  track of whether it's day or night, and going outside in
  your jammies may be a daily occurrence.

- **Mood changes:** Depression, impatience, and euphoric
  and uninhibited behavior may become more prevalent,
  leading to the person making inappropriate and even
  sexual recommendations to strangers. This stage is also
  marked by anxiety, which manifests itself most often in
  the form of following loved ones about and continually
  seeking comfort from them.

- **Suspicious minds:** This stage of dementia is
  characterized by paranoia and suspicion, which can lead
  to aggressiveness toward those who are suspected of
  stealing from the sufferer or of being out to harm him.

- **Self-care:** In this stage of dementia, people's hygiene decreases, and they need to be reminded to change their clothes, wash and shower, and brush their teeth. They may also develop incontinence, which makes keeping clean and neat even more difficult.

Identifying the Late Stage

Dementia's effects have progressed to the point that they are now severe. Sufferers at this point may be completely reliant on others for daily care and may already be in a nursing home or a care facility. Symptoms differ from person to person, but they're nearing the end of their lives.

Knowing It's the Final Chapter

At this stage, the person with dementia succumbs to the full extent of the disease's consequences, putting to rest the misconception that dementia is merely a memory problem. While there is a significant loss of memory in this stage, there is also an erosion of much of the capacity to live in any meaningful way as an independent individual, resulting in an existential loss of self.

Unfortunately, cognitive impairment isn't the only symptom of this stage of dementia; it also affects the sufferer's physical ability. Sufferers are not only unable to carry out the most basic activities of daily life, but they also become physically frail, putting them at risk of falling and making them extremely vulnerable to serious infections.

There are always exceptions to this pattern of deterioration, but any faculties that haven't already been lost or shut down for most people in the late stages of dementia begin to do so now. This shift can be seen in a variety of ways:

- Physical frailty may necessitate confinement to a wheelchair at first, and then to a bed later.

- Feeding difficulties, compounded by swallowing issues, can lead to substantial weight loss.

- While occasional moments of clear reminiscence may occur, people in this stage are more likely to have little recollection of day-to-day events, names of objects, and, most upsetting for families, names of their nearest and dearest.

- People with severe dementia may only be able to utter individual words and sounds, which are often repeated. They also lose their ability to grasp what others are saying, making meaningful interaction nearly impossible.

- Agitation and irritation are widespread, and failure to cooperate with caregivers is a common occurrence. To well-intentioned offers of assistance, people may scream, lash out with their hands and fists, pull hair, and bite. It's not uncommon for family members and spouses to find this blatant rejection of their best efforts to reach out to a loved one quite upsetting and emotionally tough to deal with.

Moving Towards the End of Life

As we sat at her mother's bedside, the daughter of one of my patients told me that she felt she'd lost her mother to dementia a long time ago and was just waiting for her body to catch up so she could begin grieving properly. This is a prevalent sentiment among a person's relatives and friends.

And I say this not only from clinical experience working with patients and their families but also from personal experience. My uncle and grandmother both suffered from various forms of dementia, and when they reached the point where it had robbed them of their minds, physical strength, and identities, it was a relief when they died.

Dementia patients in their later stages are more vulnerable to certain health problems than people of the same peer group who do not have dementia. Death can be caused by a variety of factors, including:

- Falls result in fractures, as well as poor healing and/or complications following fracture repair surgery. Stress brought on by the trauma and the experience of being in the hospital can both be lethal.

- Infections caused by bed sores, such as pneumonia, urinary tract infections, or skin infections.

- Poor nutrition and weakness cause a progressive decline in general health.

While many of the causes above are likely to expedite death, it's also very common for persons with dementia to simply give up on life and die peacefully as a result of increasing fragility.

Chapter 3

Changing The Roles

"You have Dementia. Probable Alzheimer's disease." Mum looked from the doctor's face to mine, and it occurred to her that this feeling must be what people meant when they said it was like the air was sucked out of the room.

I had seen this coming for months now. Now, this doctor was announcing a disease that would change her life. So matter-of-fact, as if the subject were heartburn. Mum watched as he scrawled a prescription and handed it past her hands and into mine.

"You can get answers from the Alzheimer's Association if you have any questions. Just go online." And just like that, the appointment was over. We walked out in silence; then stopped to schedule a three-month follow-up. Mum wondered what they would be following up on. It was up to me to ask.

Dementia impacts the patient and their family. Family connections nearly always alter as roles and duties shift and crucial decisions are made, and conflict often ensues. Maintaining strong family communication is difficult but vital while providing care.

Changing Roles

Dementia changes family roles. A spouse often feels responsible for a former partner while recognizing they've lost future aspirations. They may grow burdened managing financial and legal problems earlier handled by their spouse. This causes bitterness, desertion, and tiredness.

Adult children may become their parents' caregivers, reversing lifetime roles. As they care for a parent with dementia and their own family, they may feel exhausted and guilty. A caregiver's offspring may resent less time and attention from their parent and be bewildered or embarrassed by their grandparents' changing and unpredictable behavior.

Relationships Stressed

Caring for a dementia patient can change roles and strain family ties. Siblings and other family members may have problems embracing the person's condition and refuse to manage care, burdening the caregiver. Resentment may arise toward distant relatives who can't help as much. Distanced residents may feel ignored or invalidated. In stressful conditions, old family conflicts may reemerge, and disagreements may arise over funds and care.

Teamwork Is Important

Caregiving requires positive communication. When drafting a care plan, it's crucial to consider each family member's ideas and feelings so nobody feels left out. Sharing responsibility helps prevent primary caregiver fatigue. Family members who live far away might aid by handling finances or insurance or by contacting weekly.

Frequent communication is needed to keep everyone informed of changes and how they may affect care needs. If family issues inhibit constructive communication, a family therapist can help keep everyone connected and working together. Some families find that employing a senior care manager or home care organization reduces stress.

Caring for a member with dementia can bring families closer together. Whether positive or negative, dementia is a shared family experience.

Changing Relationships

We are social creatures, and our relationships with others shape who we are and what we value. Dementia threatens these ties, and changing positions can be emotionally taxing.

What adult child relishes becoming the parent of their father or mother? A sibling who has always looked up to a big brother may not be strong. How can a longtime partner's husband become a caregiver?

Our experience with changing roles will hinge on our attitude about them. Changes don't happen overnight, and you can probably plan shifts. Moments of sudden awareness occur, but the process is slow.

Alzheimer's doesn't make a person incompetent overnight. You left with the same individual who entered the doctor's office. You're both facing major losses, but you can console each other beforehand.

If your parent was a source of strength, you may feel adrift. As roles change, some children worry about their independence. Your father may have been distant or abusive before dementia.

As dementia develops, spouses' roles change most. Best friend? It's challenging when someone who helped make decisions, asked about your day and made you laugh can't anymore.

Dementia can affect sex and intimacy between spouses. This is worth mentioning now. You both had retirement fantasies. Grieving the life you expected is normal.

Dementia caregivers have diverse backgrounds. You're not family. My lifelong client never married or had kids, and I took her in when dementia struck. Lack of a long history can make a selection easier.

Not just the primary caregiver and dementia patient's roles alter. Friends and family will react differently to a new diagnosis. It's vital to select who, when, and what to inform.

The Alzheimer's Association interviewed dementia patients. The reactions of others to a diagnosis are often worse than the condition. Dementia patients and caregivers can't avoid this.

Older adults may remember when cancer was not discussed. If it was talked about, it was in whispers, with fear—as if the disease could hear you and come get you next. Worse, not telling the sick individual what was wrong was common.

Fast-forward to the 21st century. We talk about cancer like our diets, and the stigma is about completely gone. It moved near dementia patients, and many won't mention "the D-word" to a loved one. Hearing a friend or relative has dementia is upsetting, and fear of a similar outcome can overpower others' sadness. And we have questions: How am I expected to manage this? What's my line? Who am I? Will they remember meeting me? Why?

Close-by family and friends that don't interact might be painful. I hear the same stories: the buddy who called every Monday night, the pastor who often visited amid serious sickness, the cousin who lived a mile away and often stopped by—until dementia entered your orbit. Then, they go quiet.

Or there's the family doctor who turns away with helpless feelings of having nothing to offer. And more disappearing friends and family, with their cries of, "I can't bear to see him like that." Do they think you're glad to be there in their place?

The withdrawal of those you need at the time you need them the most is one of the biggest sources of family conflict. Old rivalries and hurt feelings often resurface in full force. While it would be great if everyone set aside their differences and rallied in a time of crisis, it's futile to ask someone for support when they can't provide it. We need outside help, and it's for our sanity.

Dementia caregiving is a journey of subtle lines, and one is acknowledging truth vs putting future sadness onto the present.

Dementia teaches us to live in the moment. This lesson is not simple. We're used to planning, worrying, and thinking forward, and dementia worsens these tendencies.

In dementia caregiving, the tendency to worry about the future can become lethal. One in six spousal caregivers don't survive the journey; they die first. The physical toll of constant worry is much to blame.

We must control our ideas for ourselves and our families. What happens if you fall? When you're tempted to put yourself last, ask yourself this.

Recognizing and appreciating changes as they occur and allowing yourself to grieve what was and is no longer help during this time of changing responsibilities.

Few approaches to change cause more pain than clinging to old patterns. The more we insist on having what has been, the harder it becomes to see the joy in what remains. And the good news is that a great deal of joy is yet to come your way.

CHANGES IN ROLES

When one family member becomes ill, roles, obligations, and expectations shift. "The worst thing is doing the checkbook," remarked one wife. We've been married for 35 years, and now I'm supposed to learn how to balance a checkbook."

"I feel like a fool cleaning ladies' underpants in the laundromat," a spouse complained.

"My father has always been the head of the household," a son commented. I don't know how I will tell him he can't drive."

"Why can't my brother pitch in and take a turn looking after Mother?" a daughter asked.

Roles differ from obligations, and it's important to understand what they mean to you and your family. Responsibilities are the roles that each family member plays. Who you are, how you are perceived, and what is expected of you are all aspects of your role. We use the term "role" to refer to a person's position in his family (for example, head of the household, mother, or "the one everyone turns to"). Roles are formed over a long period of time and are not always easy to define. Our roles are frequently symbolized by tasks. Family members recall needing to learn new tasks (doing the laundry or handling the checkbook) as well as changes in roles in the instances above (money manager, homemaker, head of the household).

When you're dealing with the various day-to-day demands of the confused person, yourself, and your family, learning a new responsibility, such as keeping the checkbook or cleaning clothes, can be challenging. Changes in roles, on the other hand, are generally more difficult to accept or adjust to. Understanding that each person's obligations change throughout time, as well as the roles and expectations of others, will aid you in comprehending personal feelings and issues that may emerge in families. It's a good idea to recall that you've dealt with position changes before and that this experience will help you adjust to new duties.

As a person's dementia advances, role changes occur in a variety of relationships. The following are four examples.

1. When a husband or wife becomes ill, their relationship changes. Some of these changes might be depressing and painful, while others can be enlightening.

Shane had been married to Sheila for fifty years when he was diagnosed with dementia. Shane had always been the leader of the household, supporting the family, paying the bills, and making the most of the major decisions, so she saw herself as someone who was constantly reliant on him. She realized she had no idea how much money they had, what insurance they had, or even how to balance a checkbook when he developed dementia. Bills were piling up, but when she confronted John about it, he screamed at her.

Sheila prepared a little turkey for his birthday and arranged an intimate luncheon where they could forget about what was going on. When she placed the electric carving knife in front of John, he screamed at her that the knife was broken and that she had damaged the turkey. She took the knife to keep the peace, only to discover that she had no idea how to carve a turkey. Shane stormed out after Sheila wept. That night, neither of them felt like eating.

Carving a turkey seemed to be the final straw for her. Shane could no longer do it, and he couldn't manage their finances; she was suddenly overwhelmed and bewildered. She had relied on him to solve difficulties throughout their marriage. She now had to learn to do the things he had always done while also dealing with his condition.

Learning new skills and responsibilities takes time and effort, and it adds to the workload you currently have. You might not want to take on new responsibilities. Few husbands want to learn how to do the laundry, and more than one has had a load of shrunken sweaters and pale pink jockey shorts before discovering that red sweaters and white underwear cannot be washed together.

A spouse who has never handled money may believe he lacks the skills to manage money and is terrified of making mistakes.

Aside from the fact that you'll have to do the task, the fact that you'll have to take it away from your spouse may signify all of the negative developments that have occurred. Mary's cutting of the turkey signified John's loss of status as the family's leader.

A spouse may eventually realize that she is alone in her difficulty since she has lost the partner with whom she shared it. Shane couldn't picture herself relying on her spouse any longer. She found herself, at the age of 60, on her own and compelled to be self-sufficient with no one to help her. It's no surprise that she felt overwhelmed by the endeavor. Learning new abilities, on the other hand, progressively provided Sheila with a sense of accomplishment. "I was shocked at myself, honestly, that I could manage things," she admitted. "It was excellent for me to learn that I could manage so effectively, even when I was upset."

Problems can appear insurmountable at times because they need you to learn new responsibilities as well as shift jobs. It's difficult to learn new skills while you're irritated and weary. You may need some practical advice for getting started with new tasks, in addition to understanding the distress that shifting jobs might create.

If you have to take over the chores, you may usually start slowly and learn as you go. However, you can avoid the aggravation of burned dinners and soiled laundry by seeking assistance. Most men and women who cook for themselves and work full-time have a variety of quick-to-prepare meals. In the store, you might even find valuable brochures or recipes.

It might be difficult to take this symbol of independence away from someone you care about. It's even worse if you're not used to handling money.

You may find it difficult to learn this new duty if you have never balanced a checkbook or paid your expenses. Even for those who despise arithmetic, managing home money is not difficult. Most banks have employees who will provide you with free advice. They will also demonstrate how to balance a checkbook. This topic is covered in books in the library. It's sometimes difficult to complete because you have to take over this role rather than the activity itself.

A list of your or the confused person's assets and debts can also be drawn out with the help of a bank or a lawyer. Sometimes a person has kept financial matters private, told no one, and now can't recall them.

Look for a driver education course geared for adults if you can't or don't want to drive and need to take over the driving responsibilities.

For driver's education and defensive driving programs for older individuals, contact the police or AARP. If you feel at ease behind the wheel, life will be much easier.

2. The relationship between a dementia-stricken dad and his adult children frequently has to shift. "Role reversal" describes the changes that occur when an adult child is forced to take on the responsibility and care of a parent.

We believe it is more accurate to describe the required changes as shifts in roles and duties, in which the adult son or daughter gradually acquires greater responsibility for a parent although the roles of parent and adult child may stay unchanged. These adjustments can be challenging. You, the adult son or daughter, may be saddened and grieved by the losses you witness in someone you like. You can feel bad about "taking command."

"I can't tell my mother she shouldn't live alone any longer; I know I should, but every time I attempt to talk to her, she makes me feel like a small child who has done something wrong."

Many of us, as adults, still believe that our parents are parents and that we, the children, are less confident, capable, and "grown-up." In some families, parents appear to retain this type of relationship with their adult offspring long after their adult sons and daughters have grown up and become self-sufficient.

Some people have had strained relationships with their parents. There may be a lot of sadness and conflict if a father hasn't been able to let his grown children feel like adults. As the parent's dementia progresses, he may appear to be demanding and manipulative of you. You may feel trapped. You may feel abused, enraged, and guilty all at once.

What you consider to be demanding may be perceived differently by the disabled individual. He could believe that with "just a little aid," he can maintain his freedom and even live alone. As he becomes aware of his decline, this may appear to be the only way he can cope with his losses.

Physically caring for a parent, such as bathing their mother or changing their father's underpants, can make adult children feel ashamed. Look for strategies to help your parent maintain his dignity while providing necessary care.

3. Dementia patients must adjust to their shifting positions in the family.

This frequently entails relinquishing some of his autonomy, authority, or leadership, which is tough for anyone. As he recognizes his abilities are decreasing, he may become disheartened. He might not be able to change or acknowledge his deterioration.

How you approach him as he grows ill will be influenced by the roles he has played in the family in the past and the type of person he is. Even if he can no longer perform the tasks he used to, you may assist him in maintaining his status as an important family member. Consult him, speak with him, and pay attention to him (even if what he says seems confused). Show him that he is still respected by your behaviors.

4. As the person with dementia's duties change, so do the expectations and roles of each family member concerning other family members. Family roles have been established for years, and your interactions and expectations of family members are founded on them. Changes frequently result in disagreements, misunderstandings, and moments when people's expectations of one another differ. Adapting to changes and dealing with

challenges, on the other hand, can bring families closer together, even if they haven't been in touch in years.

UNDERSTANDING FAMILY CONFLICTS

Division of Responsibility

"My brother doesn't have anything to do with Mom anymore," my sister continues, "and he was always her favorite." He won't even visit her. My sister and I bear the brunt of the responsibility. Because my sister's marriage is in jeopardy, I try not to leave Mom with her for long periods. As a result, I'm on my own with Mom."

The burden of caring for an incapacitated individual is sometimes not evenly distributed among family members. You might find yourself, like Mrs. Eaton, shouldering the majority of the strain of caring for someone with dementia. There are a variety of reasons why evenly dividing responsibilities is difficult. Some family members may live far away, be in bad health, be unable to contribute financially, or have issues with their children or marriage.

Families may accept stereotypes about who should help without evaluating what is best for them. According to one notion, daughters (and daughters-in-law) are "expected" to look after the sick. However, the daughter or daughter-in-law may already be overburdened and unable to handle this responsibility. She may have young children or work full-time, and perhaps she is a single mother or father.

Even if we aren't conscious of them, long-established roles, obligations, and mutual expectations within the family can play an essential role in defining who is responsible for the impaired individual.

As an example,

"I was raised by my mother; now I must look after her."

"She was a good wife, and she would have done the same for me," says the narrator.

"I married him at a late age." What is my responsibility, and what is his children's responsibility?"

"He was always harsh with me, abandoned my mother when I was ten, and left all of his money to some charity. I'm not sure how much I owe him."

Understanding Family Conflicts

Expectations aren't always logical and may not be founded on the most realistic or equitable arrangement. The illness crisis sometimes exacerbates long-standing family arguments, resentments, or conflicts.

Because it is difficult for them to grasp the reality of the impaired person's sickness, family members may not be able to aid as much as they could.

Sometimes it's too much for a person to handle or face this condition. It's difficult to watch a loved one deteriorate, as you know. Family members who do not have the responsibility of daily care are sometimes reluctant to visit because the decline saddens them. Others in the family, on the other hand, may interpret this as abandoning the ailing relative.

Occasionally, one family member takes on the majority of the caregiving responsibilities. He is not allowed to tell other family members how horrible things are. He may not want to bother them, or he may not truly desire their assistance.

"I fear to call on my sons," Mr. Newman admits. They are willing to assist, but they also have jobs and families."

Frequently, you and other family members have strong and divergent opinions about how things should be done. This occurs occasionally because not all family members understand what is wrong with the dementia patient, why he acts the way he does, or what to expect in the future.

Family members who do not share the day-to-day experience of living with a person with dementia may be judgmental or unsympathetic because they do not understand what it is like. It's difficult for outsiders to comprehend how exhausting the everyday load of ongoing care may be. People often have no idea how you're feeling unless you tell them.

A family member may occasionally obstruct your efforts to seek outside assistance. If this occurs, demand that a family member assists in the care of the disabled individual so that you can rest. If the family member lives out of town, invite him to join a support group in his area or volunteer at a dementia program so that he can better appreciate what you're going through. In the end, the family must recognize that the person who is responsible for the majority of the care should make the final decision on whether to use day care, in-home care, or a nursing facility. When everyone is educated about what resources are available and how much they will cost, there are fewer misconceptions.

Marriage

When the sick person is a parent or in-law, it's crucial to think about how his illness may affect your marriage. It's not always easy to keep a good marriage going, and caring for someone with a dementing illness can make it even more challenging. It could entail additional financial strains and less time to converse, socialize, and make love. It could mean spending more time with your in-laws, having more things to argue about, being exhausted all the time, or neglecting your children. It may entail having to live with a difficult, disagreeable, and seemingly demanding dementia patient.

It's difficult to watch someone develop dementia. Normally, a person could question if his spouse will become like his disabled in-law and if he'll have to go through this again.

A son or daughter might easily become split between the requirements of an ailing parent, the expectations of siblings (or the other parent), and the wants and demands of a spouse and children.

It's all too easy to vent our frustrations or exhaustion on the people we love and trust the most: our spouse and children.

A spouse of a parent with a disability may likewise cause issues. He or she may be upset, critical, or unwell, or he or she may even abandon his or her disabled partner. Such issues can exacerbate strain in your marriage and should be discussed with everyone concerned if at all possible. It is sometimes easier if a son or a daughter initiates a solution with his or her own family.

Amid stress and difficulties, a healthy relationship can survive for a while, but we believe the husband and wife must find time and energy for each other—to talk, to get away, and to enjoy their relationship in the ways that they have always done.

MANAGING CHANGES IN ROLE AND FAMILY CONFLICT

When family members disagree, or when the majority of the load falls on one person, it exacerbates the issues you're dealing with. Caring for a chronically ill person is frequently too much for one person to handle. It is critical that you have others to assist you— to provide you with "time off" from continual care, encouragement and support, work assistance, and financial responsibility sharing.

It's not a good idea to let your animosity simmer if you're getting criticism or not enough aid from your family. It may be up to you to take the initiative in your family to make changes. This can be tough to do when families are at odds or when long-standing problems get in the way.

How do you deal with the frequently complex and difficult role shifts brought on by a chronic, debilitating illness? To begin, acknowledge that these are features of family connections. Knowing that family responsibilities are complex, frequently unacknowledged and that changes can be difficult will help you feel less anxious and overwhelmed. Recognize that particular activities may be symbolic of essential family duties and that it is the transition in the role, not the exact issue, that may be unpleasant.

Learn everything you can about the condition. What family members think is accurate about the condition has an impact on how much assistance they supply and whether or not there will be arguments about how to care for the disabled person. Local Alzheimer's Association meetings can be attended by family members who live out of town.

Consider the distinctions between the responsibilities or tasks that an impaired person may be forced to relinquish and the positions that he may be able to keep. While John's condition prevents him from carving a turkey or making many decisions, his position as Mary's adored and beloved husband may continue.

Determine what the disabled person can still perform and what is too tough for him. Of course, one wants a person to be as self-sufficient as possible, but unrealistic expectations can make him upset and unhappy. (Expectations about how well he can function can originate from others, but they can also arise from the handicapped individual themselves.) If he is unable to complete a task alone, attempt to simplify it so that he can do a portion of it.

Recognize that position transitions are continuous processes rather than one-time events. You may need to continue to take on more responsibilities as your sickness advances. You'll probably relive some of the sensations of despair and being overwhelmed by your job each time. In the case of a chronic illness, this is a normal part of the grieving process.

Talk to other families about your experience. One of the benefits of family support groups is this. It may be reassuring to read that other families have faced similar challenges. Laugh a little at yourself. Try to find the humor in the situation if you've just burned dinner or hacked up a turkey. When the family of dementia patients gathers together, they often cry and laugh over their experiences.

Look for methods to assist one another. When a wife is responsible for most of the daily care for an ailing parent, she may be in desperate need of her husband's assistance with odd duties like housework or waiting with the parent while she goes out. She will undoubtedly require his love and encouragement, as well as his assistance with the rest of the family.

You may reach a point where the scope and expectations of your caregiving job are too much for you to handle. You must be able to recognize this and take action.

When the time comes, you and the Person with Dementia as a Family make alternate arrangements. Your decision-making responsibilities may eventually include deciding to relinquish your role as the primary caregiver.

A Family Conference

A family conference, we believe, is one of the most effective strategies to assist families in coping. Hold a family gathering, with the support of a counselor or a physician if necessary, to discuss issues and develop plans. You can make firm decisions about how much support or money each person will provide if you work together.

There are certain ground principles for a family conference that you may offer at the outset: everyone (including children who will be affected by the decision) must attend, each person must speak freely, and everyone must listen to what the others have to say (even if they disagree).

If family members differ about what is wrong with the confused, forgetful person or how to manage his care, giving other family members this book and other written resources about the disease, or asking the doctor to speak with them, may be helpful. It's astonishing how often this helps to alleviate family conflicts.

When you get together, here are some questions to ask each other. What exactly are the issues? Now, who is doing what? What must be done, and who is capable of doing it? What can you do to assist each other? What does it mean for each of you as a result of these changes? The following are some of the practical issues that may need to be addressed: Who will be in charge of daily care? Does this imply a loss of privacy? You're not inviting friends over? Not being able to take a vacation because you can't afford it? Is this to say that because their parents will be preoccupied with the Alzheimer's patient, they will expect their children to act more maturely? Who will decide whether or not to admit a parent to a nursing home?

Who Will Be in Charge of the Person's Funds?

What will a well-spouse of an impaired person's position in the family be if he or she moves into a son's or daughter's house with the impaired person? Is she going to be in charge of the grandchildren? Will the kitchen be used by two people? While having a larger family can be beneficial, it can also lead to conflict. Anticipating and discussing potential areas of dispute ahead of time can make things go more smoothly.

It's also vital to discuss a few more practical areas where family relationships can go wrong. When a loved one is unwell, it may seem insensitive to think about money or inheritance, yet financial concerns and doubts about who will inherit an inheritance are real—if frequently hidden—factors in assessing responsibility for a family member. They can be the source of a lot of resentment. Money is something that needs to be spoken about openly. Consider the following inquiries.

1. Is everyone aware of the amount of money and inheritance available? "Dad has that stock he acquired twenty years ago, he

owns his house, and he has his Social Security," one son thinks frequently. He should be perfectly at ease." The second son, who is caring for his father, is well aware that "the house needs a new roof and a new furnace," that "old mining stock is worthless," and that "he gets barely enough money from Social Security and I have to pay for his medicine out of my own pocket."

2. Is there a desire to succeed? Is there anyone who knows or suspects he has been shortchanged in his will? Do some family members believe that others are lusting for inherited money, property, or personal belongings? This is not uncommon, and it is best dealt with when it is addressed directly. Hidden resentments can smolder and manifest as disagreements over the person's daily care.

3. How much does it cost to care for a dementia patient, and who is responsible for paying the bills? There are many "hidden" costs to consider when caring for a person at home: special foods, medication, special door latches, a sitter, transportation, another bed and dresser on the ground floor, grab bars for the bathroom, and perhaps the cost of a spouse not working to care for the confused person.

4. Does everyone understand how much it costs to care for a dementia patient in a nursing home, and who is legally accountable for those expenditures?

When a daughter says, "Mother has to put Dad in a nursing home," she may not realize that she is making a financial mistake.

5. Do some family members believe that money has been given unequally in the past? As an example,

"Dad paid for my brother's college education and the down payment on his house." "But now that my brother won't take him, I'm stuck with the job—and the cost—of caring for him."

"There's no way you'll bring my family together to talk about that," families may say. My brother will not even talk about it over the phone. And if we did get together, it would be a major brawl." You may be discouraged if you believe your family is like this. Despite the fact that you require your family's assistance, you may feel trapped because you believe your family will not assist you. It is not uncommon for families to seek the assistance of a third party—a counselor, minister, or social worker—to help them work through their issues and reach equitable agreements.

As members of a family, you and the person with dementia can listen objectively and assist the family in keeping the conversation focused on the issues at hand rather than drifting off into old arguments. Your doctor, a social worker, or a counselor may be able to intervene on your behalf and persuade everyone involved to hold a family meeting to discuss issues that are important to all of them. A family lawyer may be able to assist you. If you need legal assistance, choose an attorney who is really interested in resolving problems rather than assisting you in bringing a lawsuit against your own family. If a family is having difficulties and you seek assistance from a third party, the first item of discussion may be to agree that the third party will not take sides with any one person.

You require the support of your family. Now is a great time to put old grudges aside for the sake of the disabled individual. If your family is unable to reconcile all of your differences, perhaps you can identify one or two points of agreement in a discussion. Everyone will be encouraged, and the next debate will be easier.

When You Live in the Countryside

"My father looks after my mother." They live nearly a thousand miles away, and it's difficult for me to see them frequently. Dad doesn't seem to tell me how horrible things are. It's simply so difficult being so far away: you feel guilty and powerless."

"I can't say anything because I'm just the daughter-in-law." They haven't received a satisfactory diagnosis. They continue to visit their old family doctor. I'm concerned that she's suffering from another ailment. But they always pretend they didn't hear me when I make a suggestion."

Special issues arise when the confused person and the person who provides daily care do not live in the same neighborhood. Long-distance family members are equally as concerned as those who live close by, and they frequently feel frustrated and powerless. They are concerned that they do not understand what is going on, that the caregiver has not received the most accurate diagnosis, or that the caregiver should act differently. They may feel guilty for not being able to be with their family when they are needed.

If you don't see someone very often, it can be tough to comprehend the severity of their restrictions at first. The shock of later realizing how a person has deteriorated can be devastating.

The single most significant contribution you can make to the disabled family member is your support of the individual who provides daily care. Dementia frequently persists for a long time. You must establish long-term family cooperation. If the person who provides daily care initially rejects your suggestions, she may eventually accept them.

Allow the regular caregiver to take a break. Consider having the impaired person stay with you for a few weeks, or go stay with the impaired person while the usual caregiver is away. Moving an impaired person to a new home can be upsetting, but it can also serve as a "vacation" for both the impaired person and the caregiver, especially early in a dementing illness.

If you live a long distance away from the person with dementia, consider sending videotapes or a digital movie of yourself, hiring a sitter so that the caregiver can go out, sending a card to the person with dementia every day, or calling the person at the same time every day. Just say "Hello" for a minute; don't expect the person to be able to hold a long conversation.

What Can You Do to Assist If You Are Not the Primary Caregiver?

Families in the United States do not abandon their senior members and do not forsake each other. Despite their flaws, families can usually work out their differences and stick together for the long haul.

There are numerous activities that family members can participate in. One caregiver may require a daily phone call; another may require a sitter so he can go out once a week; another may require someone to come over on short notice when things become rough; yet another may simply require a shoulder to cry on.

- Maintain a close relationship. Keep lines of communication open with the caregiver. This will allow you to recognize when the caregiver requires further assistance. When caregivers feel fully supported by their family, they manage better and endure less stress. It's not just how much help caregivers get that helps them deal better; it's also how well they feel supported.

- Don't criticize. The majority of the time, criticism does not result in positive change.

- Nobody enjoys being chastised. Many of us tend to dismiss criticism. If you feel compelled to speak up, be sure your critique is valid. Are you certain you comprehend the situation if you don't live nearby?

- Recognize that the primary caregiver must make that ultimate decision. Although you can offer assistance and advice, the person who provides daily care must make decisions such as whether or not she can employ outside aid and whether or not she can continue to provide care.

- Assume responsibility for locating assistance. Caregivers
  are frequently overwhelmed to the point where they are
  unable to find a sitter or a daycare facility, improved
  medical treatment, supportive equipment, or assistance
  for themselves. Even locating a place to rest can include
  making phone calls. Take on this task and urge your
  relative to seek respite care by being nice and sympathetic

- Keep yourself up to date. You'll be able to help the most
  if you understand both the sickness and what your
  family's caregiver is going through. There are good books
  that describe dementia and publications written by
  carers. Attend meetings of local family support groups.
  You might meet other long-distance relatives, and you
  might hear from the main caregivers what their long-
  distance relatives did to help them the most. Do not
  succumb to the desire to disregard the issue. Because
  these diseases are so deadly, the entire family must band
  together.

- Contact the ill person's doctor and others who have
  assessed him. Ask direct inquiries if they are willing. If
  you have doubts about the diagnosis, the adequacy of the
  assessment, or the disease's anticipated trajectory, get
  advice from clinicians who are familiar with the person

- Take over the responsibilities that the confused individual
  used to have. Bring over a home-cooked supper, balance
  the checkbook, and take the automobile to the mechanic.

- Allow the caregiver to take a break. For a weekend, a
  week, or a few days, look after your relative while the
  primary caregiver is away. Before you begin, many
  Alzheimer's Association chapters will teach you the
  fundamentals of caregiving. Not only will the caregiver

benefit from the break, but it will also bring you and the caregiver closer together.

- Take walks, go out to dinner, play with the cat together, or go window shopping to do things that are soothing and enjoyable for the handicapped person.

If you are unable to help on your own, seek assistance. Adult day care and sitter care are available in many places. You can also hire someone to do your shopping, fix your car, or locate resources.

Your Job and Caregiving

Many caregivers work full- or part-time while caring for a person with dementia. The dual duties of caring for a family and working can be exhausting. When there is an issue with the disabled individual, some caretakers must take time off from work. When there is no other option, caregivers must sometimes leave the befuddled person alone, even if it is not safe. Even caregivers who enlist the help of a good adult daycare facility or a dependable sitter encounter additional challenges. When a person with dementia is awake and active late at night, for example, the caregiver loses sleep.

If you're considering quitting your career to care for a loved one full-time, weigh your options carefully. Many caregivers have reported feeling more stressed and unhappy after quitting their jobs. Full-time caregiving may require you to put up with the person's irritating behavior all of the time, and you may feel more lonely and stuck than you did when you could leave the house and go to work. Leaving a job usually entails a large financial loss. It could imply putting your career on hold and failing to stay current in your field. It can be challenging to return to work after several years of caregiving. Is there going to be a vacancy? Will you lose your benefits or seniority?

Discuss your choices with your employer before deciding to leave. Is it possible to work with more flexible hours? Is it possible for you to split the work? Is it feasible to take a paid or unpaid leave of absence? Some caring daughters and sons discover that a good nursing home is a better option for them and the dementia patient.

Your Children

Having children at home might present unique challenges during this time. Because they, too, have a bond with the dementia patient, they may have complex thoughts about their condition and unexpressed questions about what's happening. This is not unusual; parents frequently worry about the impact on their children of exposure to someone with dementia. It's sometimes difficult or awkward to talk to a child about the sometimes strange, sometimes alarming behavior of the afflicted parent or grandparent. Parents are sometimes concerned that their children will pick up bad habits from dementia patients.

The majority of the time, children are aware of what is going on. They are keen observers who, even when things are kept hidden from them, can detect when something isn't quite right. Children, fortunately, are remarkably resilient. Even tiny children can benefit from an honest explanation of what is occurring to a person with dementia in a language they understand. This makes them less frightened. Assure youngsters that this illness is not contagious like the flu and that neither they nor their parents are at risk of contracting it. Tell the child that nothing he did contributed to his sickness. Sometimes children subconsciously believe they are to blame for their family's misfortunes.

When discussing dementia with a child, be honest, be specific and don't act like it's something terrible or to be afraid of. Use words like this:

"Grandma has a sickness that causes her to act like she does. She doesn't realize it. It's scary sometimes, but she doesn't mean it." Make sure you let the child know that "None of us will be like Grandma. You can't catch this like a cold. What's happening is that parts of Grandma's brain are very sick. She won't get better.

"You know how hard it was when you were trying to learn to do your buttons or tie your shoes? Grandma is like that, except she's not learning, she's forgetting. And she acts mad sometimes, because she's scared. But the important thing to remember is that Grandma is always going to love you because she always has. Even if she forgets, she still loves. So we need to love her back and let her know she doesn't have to be scared."

It is normally better to actively involve youngsters in what is going on in the family and even find ways for them to contribute. Small toddlers often have a special bond with handicapped, confused individuals and can form special and loving ties with them. Make an environment where the child feels free to ask you questions and express his feelings.

Remember that children experience loss and grief as well, yet they may be able to enjoy a handicapped person's youthful behaviors without feeling sad. The more at ease you are with your knowledge of this illness, the easier it will be to explain it to your child.

Children may want assistance in deciding what to say to peers who tease them about a "funny" parent or grandparent. If you don't make a considerable deal out of it and the child is getting adequate love and attention, youngsters would rarely emulate the negative behaviors of a person with dementia for long. Explain to the child (usually multiple times) that his parent or grandparent has a condition and cannot control his conduct, but that the youngster can and is expected to do so.

Preparing and Teaching Young Children What to Expect

Children who don't understand the situation are sometimes concerned that something they did or might do will aggravate the situation. It is critical to discuss these concerns with the young child and to reassure him or her. Don't make the mistake of assuming you know what a child is thinking, and realize that children, even small children, do feel pity, sadness, and sympathy.

With that in mind, make sure you discuss what is going on with your kids regularly. Even long after the confused person has gone to a nursing facility or has passed, the impact of this sickness lingers. Be open to the children's questions and be ready to continue the conversation.

Attempt to include all of the children in the person's care on an equal basis. Children may find it difficult to be relied upon or may feel excluded. They gain a sense of responsibility by sharing in caring.

The parent closest to the dementia patient must be mindful of the children's emotions and how her sadness and distress may be impacting them. Parents can become so consumed by their own problems that they forget about their children's needs. Their actions can be as distressing to the kids as the illness itself.

When there are children at home, the most serious issue is that the parent's time and energy are divided between the handicapped person and the children, with never enough time or energy for both. To deal with this double burden, you'll need all the aid you can get—help from the rest of the family, community resources, and time—to refill your emotional and physical energies. You can be divided between neglecting your children and neglecting a "childish" or demanding dementia patient.

As the person's condition deteriorates, so will your predicament. The deteriorating person may require increasing amounts of care and may be so disruptive that children are unable to feel safe at home. You might not have the physical or emotional energy to care for children or teenagers, let alone a dementia patient. As a result of the person's disease, children growing up in such a setting may suffer.

To provide a better home environment for the children, you may have to make the difficult decision to place the dementia patient in a nursing home. If you find yourself in this situation, you and your children should talk about what to do and what each of your options means to each family member. "We'll have less money for movies, but we won't have Dad screaming at us all night." "We'll have to move and change schools, but I'll be able to bring my friends home." Avoid giving the impression that the placement is solely based on their requirements. Let them know that you made the decision because it was the greatest thing for the entire family.

Chapter 4

Providing Care During The Onset Stage

You'll learn how to be and become an effective caregiver for someone who has Alzheimer's disease (AD) in its early stages, with an emphasis on how to cope with the diagnosis and make lifestyle changes. Some caretakers may become parental in this situation, wanting to step in and make decisions for the individual even if he or she still has the ability to do so. In all cases, however, it is critical for both the person experiencing cognitive changes and the caregiver to collaborate, which means that issues are discussed and decisions are made together.

The Experience of Loss

Cognitive impairment develops slowly in people with Alzheimer's disease and it is typically undetected until it begins to interfere with everyday life. Individuals who notice every memory loss and are concerned about it (because they remember everything they forgot!) are often more stressed than those who are genuinely impaired. Other diseases, such as a major operation, a minor stroke, or a head injury, might cause mild cognitive impairment to appear suddenly. Both the person experiencing cognitive changes and the caregiver may feel a sense of loss, dread, and uncertainty about the future in each scenario.

It's not difficult to imagine what it's like to have dementia. We've all had the "tip-of-the-tongue" experience, where we can't quite recall the name of something despite its familiarity. Imagine having similar experiences numerous times a day—for names, people, places, and recent events—and you'll have a sense of what it's like to suffer from moderate symptoms. Many people with dementia report their symptoms as missing portions of the day, recent experiences, and once-familiar objects. It can be aggravating, but it is not incapacitating, and with a few minor adjustments, the person can lead a reasonably normal life. Many people will be frightened and unhappy as a result of the changes and may withdraw from social situations out of embarrassment or to hide the changes from others. There are occasions when people have unpleasant experiences, such as when friends or family members question or criticize them about a memory loss in an insensitive way. In such conditions, mild symptoms might deteriorate into a life-threatening crisis.

Given the challenges and frustrations that a person with mild cognitive impairment faces, there are a few basic measures that can help. First, obtain a thorough evaluation so that you and your partner both understand what's going on, what kind of impairment is there, and what can be done. Second, exercise patience. Do not remind the person of what he or she is forgetting, and do not tease or become upset with him or her. Instead, offer assistance when the person requires it. Concentrate on your advantages: Memory lapses do not necessarily imply that other cognitive abilities are compromised. Finally, maintain a positive outlook and let the individual know that he or she is appreciated as a person, not for what they can recall. There are always ways to improve, slow down, or at the very least stabilize cognitive changes. There are numerous resources available to assist you. There are family and friends that will understand and help.

Giving care can be a huge load, resulting in increased stress, medical issues, and sadness. Caregivers who look after themselves as well as the person they are caring for are healthier and more effective.

Overcoming Resistance

Some people who are experiencing early-stage symptoms hesitate to see a doctor. This is not uncommon, and it might be caused by a fear of a diagnosis, denial, or a lack of understanding of the situation. Individuals may be concerned that if they are diagnosed with dementia, they will lose their capacity to work or participate in activities that demand critical decision-making, support their livelihood, or have significant personal importance. Caregivers sometimes join forces with them to prevent an evaluation because they share similar worries, denial, or lack of awareness, or they are afraid of losing some sort of dependence on the individual (e.g., the affected person does all of the driving or manages key household affairs). When you consider that many doctors never inquire about memory problems, it's no surprise that diagnosis and therapy can take years.

When confronted with such opposition, it's critical to underline the significance of early diagnosis and the dangers of delaying. There is greater damage done and less chance of improvement from treatment when reversible causes of cognitive impairment continue. Undiagnosed people are more likely to make poor medical, financial, and other decisions and can be exploited or mistreated as a result. They can also suffer from untreated medical and psychological disorders, as well as damage. These difficulties should be enough to persuade both the caregiver and the affected person to seek medical help.

If someone refuses to see a memory specialist, have them see a trusted doctor instead, but make sure you either accompany them to the appointment or speak with the doctor beforehand to share your concerns. Assure the client that the purpose is to evaluate for cognitive problems and possible causes in the same way that you would any other medical concern. Limit the conversation to the evaluation and avoid catastrophizing the situation by discussing serious diagnoses and possible lifestyle adjustments. You may need to be persistent with people who refuse to even see their doctor. In certain cases, try to narrow the focus even further to simply speaking with the doctor about how memory and cognition might be assessed.

Refusing to take drugs, not attending follow-up appointments or having particular tests performed, limiting driving and other high-risk activities, or making specific lifestyle adjustments are all examples of resistance. When someone just refuses to help or actively sabotages your attempts, it can be quite frustrating. You sometimes have to back off and give it time with any signs at this early stage, hoping that the person would eventually come around. You may have to approach the person at a different time. You may need to make concessions or compromises from time to time, selecting and choosing the most essential battles while ignoring others. While pushing an agenda to help the person manage cognitive limitations, you must always respect his or her privacy, dignity, and liberty. At this point, obtaining legal guardianship is frequently impossible and would likely harm your connection with the person. Finally, you will be best served if you can engage the assistance of trusted family members as well as specialists who deal with dementia on a daily basis. Other carers and caregiver resources may be able to offer advice.

Discussing Diagnosis

Doctors didn't always tell patients about serious medical diagnoses in the not-too-distant past. The word cancer was whispered or never used, and vital diagnoses were withheld from those deemed too fragile to handle the news. Today, the terms Alzheimer's disease and dementia conjure up a lot of the same anxiety, and caregivers are sometimes hesitant to even bring it up. These anxieties are understandable, however clinical experience and studies have demonstrated that patients do not have catastrophic reactions to learning of dementia diagnosis, and they do not go into depression as a result. In fact, for many people, having a name for their problems and a plan to deal with them is a relief.

It's never a good idea to dismiss, ignore, or wish away signs of cognitive impairment. Changes in memory and other cognitive skills, like significant changes in blood pressure and sugar levels, can be key warning signals of a medical or mental issue that needs to be recognized and treated. Early intervention, as emphasized throughout this book, offers the best chance of halting, slowing, or even reversing symptoms.

Even with a thorough examination, there may be some uncertainty about the precise diagnosis and course of treatment, especially in the early stages. It's difficult to predict the future when you don't know whether or how the condition will progress, which can cause a lot of anxiety and even despair. Unfortunately, even with a comprehensive workup, it is often impossible to know the exact diagnosis early on. However, it is possible to clearly define the issues, begin treatment, and start putting resources in place. There are a number of things that can be done to improve the situation and possibly slow down the progression, including becoming more educated about it, gathering resources, beginning a brain-healthy lifestyle, mobilizing family and friends, participating in research, and improving physical and mental health. Regardless of which diagnosis becomes more certain over time, all of these activities will provide a sense of control and hope, as well as aid to move things forward.

Get a Second Opinion

The majority of early-stage Alzheimer's disease diagnoses are made by primary care doctors, often without a thorough examination. Even if a specialist has completed a thorough examination, it is reasonable to seek a second opinion. This is due to a few factors. First, if the original workup did not include a comprehensive medical and psychiatric history, neuropsychological testing, a recent brain scan, or a mental status examination, something may have been missed. Important factors like alcohol abuse, depression, adult attention deficit disorder, bipolar disorder, and personality disorders that can mimic symptoms in later life are frequently overlooked by doctors. Another reason to seek a second opinion is to locate a physician with whom you can establish a solid working relationship and who can effectively manage your disease over time. Because they have social workers on staff, caregiver training, and support programs, memory centers are perfect.

Work-Related Issues

Many people begin to experience cognitive decline while they are still working, which can have serious consequences. How comfortable would you be if your anesthesiologist, your tax preparer, or the bus driver for your child or grandchild had memory problems? These scenarios demonstrate how crucial it is to obtain a thorough evaluation as soon as possible to determine the extent of the impairment and its impact on the job. Changes in mood and behavior, such as depression, apathy, or impulsivity, may also need to be taken into account. Following the completion of this baseline assessment, the person with the impairment and their caregiver must collaborate with relevant professionals to develop a plan of action to address the following issues:

Is there a chance that others will suffer physical, psychological, or financial harm as a result of your actions? If this is the case, immediate job changes or retirement should be considered. Putting the lives or livelihoods of others in jeopardy is unethical. Furthermore, injuring others could result in disastrous legal and financial ramifications if the offender is willfully endangering others. If a business or practice is perceived to be in danger, patients, clients, and others will flee. This is especially problematic for someone who runs their own company. Switching to a less hazardous role or hiring an assistant or partner to provide reminders or review work are some logical job modifications short of retirement.

Have you observed any other symptoms of cognitive impairment? If this is the case, there will undoubtedly be some explaining to do, but this could result in a slew of issues. If the person works for a corporation, it's better to keep any disclosures to the appropriate human resources person at first, and then follow their advice. They can assist the individual in crafting and directing any necessary disclosures. For smaller or solo businesses, the risk of disclosing cognitive issues may argue for bringing in a partner to take over daily responsibilities and eliminate the potential for serious errors.

Hopefully, before the commencement of issues, estate planning, wills, advance directives, and disability insurance have all been addressed. If not, you should seek legal advice to have these matters examined and resolved.

Lifestyle Modification

Mild cognitive impairment and early-stage dementia can cause impairment in a variety of skills to differing degrees, and this pattern can assist establish the lifestyle changes that are required. A person with primarily short-term memory changes, for example, will need to use memory aids such as calendars and reminder notes, as well as have caregivers remind and prompt him or her, whereas someone with more severe visuospatial impairment will require assistance getting to places and then navigating around. Mood and behavior changes will necessitate psychological or psychiatric intervention, such as talk therapy. More daily activities may help with apathy or motivation loss. Individuals always perform better when they are involved in important, engaging activities, which boost attention, concentration, motivation, and mood, in my experience.

Ask yourself the following questions to figure out what lifestyle changes you should think about:

Has the person, when alone, done anything that could put themselves or others in danger, such as leaving the stove on, taking the wrong dose of medication or missing doses, or forgetting to turn off the water? If such occurrences have occurred, greater supervision and check-ins during the day are required. Here are a few recommendations:

- Check all fire alarms, fire extinguishers, carbon monoxide detectors, and security alarms for functionality.
- If the person is alone at home, have frequent phone check-ins.
- If necessary, have a friend or neighbor check in on the person.
- Consider a security system with cameras that can be viewed from a cell phone or computer.
- Have a visiting nurse or a caregiver set up a labeled pillbox or electronic distribution device for drugs ahead of time.

Has the person been in a lot of accidents or had a lot of falls? Have any household objects been harmed as a result of abuse? If that's the case, consider the following:

- Ensure that any hearing or vision impairments have been recognized and corrected or compensated for, such as cleaning ear canals and replacing hearing aid batteries, or having eyesight checked regularly to update prescription glasses.

- Address balance, walking, coordination, tremor, sensory ability, and strength-related neurological issues. There are occasions when pharmaceutical or disease management difficulties must be addressed, such as addressing low blood sugar or avoiding taking too many sleeping pills. It is sometimes necessary to use assistive devices such as canes or walkers.

- Determine if the individual consumes excessive amounts of alcohol. This can cause damage by impairing balance, sleep, and judgment. Even excessive water consumption can result in urinary incontinence and low salt levels in the body.

Is there any evidence of weight loss? Do you find yourself sleeping a lot during the day? Is there a lack of energy? If that's the case, consider the following:

- Make sure there's enough food on hand and that it's ready to eat. You may need to prepare and store easy-to-make meals ahead of time, or arrange for Meals on Wheels.

- Look into untreated pain, particularly dental pain that may be affecting your appetite, sleep, or both.

- Make an appointment with the person's primary care physician for a comprehensive examination and a review of all medications and supplements he or she is taking.

- Has the person become disoriented while walking or driving? Consider the following if your visuospatial abilities or recognition of familiar places are impaired:

- Don't leave the person alone in strange settings. Have a companion or at the very least have point-to-point connections.

- Make sure the person has a cell phone with a navigation app and a way to contact the caregiver. Cell phones that have a tracking app can also be handy.

- Consider driving only during the day, in excellent weather, and to familiar destinations.

- Consider having a driving evaluation to see if the person is even capable of driving.

Individuals with cognitive changes and their caregivers must re examine whether the living environment is sufficiently secured and modified to accommodate the cognitive losses as more of these safety issues arise. Additional household assistance may be required.

Relationship Issues

When one partner in a relationship experiences a cognitive decline, the entire relationship changes, owing in part to what it was like before. A person with short-term memory loss or other cognitive limitations will inevitably become more reliant on others, necessitating the hiring of a caregiver. Thus, if the person who is having difficulty is not used to being dependent on others and resists or resents it, the very fact of needing aid can become a source of conflict. The caregiver, on the other hand, may not want to take on these new obligations, may not know what to do, or may not feel confident doing so. The caregiver may have been reliant on the impaired person for key tasks such as driving, earning an income, managing finances, and maintaining the home, and now must take on previously unfamiliar or unwelcome responsibilities.

Adult children who need to be involved can create a whole new set of problems if their parents do not communicate or interact well with them. Caregivers may also have conflicts with one another, such as when one sibling lives closest to the patient and must shoulder a greater share of the burden, or when there are disagreements about lifestyle choices or how to provide care. When care needs go unmet, avoidance can be an effective defense mechanism for coping with anxiety and sadness over an impaired parent, but it can lead to major problems.

The best time to address family dynamics is at the start of dementia. Here are a few of the most important questions to ask, along with some helpful hints:

Who is the primary caregiver in your family? The most prevalent caretakers are older female spouses or partners, followed by elder daughters. Husbands, sons, and daughters-in-law, on the other hand, are frequently caretakers. The primary caregiver is the one who lives with the affected person, although he or she will eventually require assistance in all areas, especially if he or she is elderly and suffering from physical frailty, acute or chronic medical or psychological difficulties, or cognitive impairment. The primary caregiver should compile a list of the areas in which he or she needs help and enlist other caregivers willing and able to pitch in.

Are there pre-existing disagreements among potential caregivers and/or family members? Sometimes the spouse is from a prior marriage and does not get along with the children from that marriage. Children may have a lengthy history of conflict with their parents or be estranged from them and have no contact with them. Cousins, neighbors, or friends are sometimes involved since they reside close by, as opposed to children who live far away, but the children do not fully trust them. There are times when children's thoughts or beliefs differ from those of the caregiver parent.

The affected person can suffer tremendously in any of these scenarios because caregivers and other concerned parties conflict with one another, sometimes to the point of legal action. A memory center's main care doctor, social worker, care manager, or clinician cannot play King Solomon and resolve these issues, but they can make important independent recommendations or act as a third party to assist in the assumption or location of specific caring obligations. All potential caregivers, involved family, and others should meet with the affected person to the best of their abilities and distribute caregiving responsibilities as fairly as possible. Find a professional who can act as an arbitrator if this isn't possible. Ask for advice from an accountant, financial planner, or eldercare attorney to sort out critical legal or financial difficulties.

Have you addressed any significant legal issues so far? Designating health care proxies, powers of attorney and estate planning are all important decisions that can help avoid future conflicts.

Is a member of your family putting up roadblocks? Unfortunately, caregivers may have to deal with one or more family members who are opposed to using common sense to manage NCDs. These people might advise against hiring home health aides, taking anti-anxiety meds, or making necessary house renovations, for example. When one family member is completely opposed to the use of medications, vaccines, or psychiatric interventions, or believes in alternative medical or natural approaches, ideological beliefs can arise. Financial motivations are frequently concealed under reluctance, such as not wanting parents to spend a prospective inheritance or not wanting one sister who is the primary carer to receive an amount that would be considered excessive. Keeping the impaired person away from other family members or getting the impaired person to sign legal documents giving them inappropriate control over finances, transferring property to them, or changing wills to exclude others from inheriting money or property are all examples of caregivers causing problems. All caregivers and family members should be aware that such behaviors can result in serious consequences, such as criminal charges for exploitation and abuse, as well as legal issues ranging from improper financial transactions to lawsuits filed by siblings.

In the end, the person who is harmed is the one who suffers the most. To all caregivers and family members, I offer the following words of wisdom: Gather now, while the affected person is still able to participate, to work out fair arrangements for caregiving responsibilities as well as all legal and financial issues. To make major medical decisions, one designated caregiver is required, and it is preferable to have someone who is not so ideological as to exclude mainstream approaches.

Are there any lingering marital or family issues? If this is the case, couples or family therapy may be beneficial, especially if the affected person is still able to engage fully. Having the opportunity to vent in front of a neutral third party who has received therapeutic training can be extremely beneficial, as it can help the person clarify where the conflict is and what can be done to improve or resolve it.

Adult children can sometimes disengage from supporting caregivers who are spouses because they are fearful of or in denial about their parent's neurocognitive disease (NCD). It's best to be clear about what you need them to do in those situations, rather than bringing up the issue of diagnosis or disease progression. If a parent has a progressive NCD, the adult children will have to deal with the severe changes in their parents sooner or later. You may have to let them get there on their own, but that doesn't rule out enlisting their assistance.

Adult children of impaired parents will likely be unable to serve as full-time caregivers due to their own responsibilities at home or work. It can be physically, emotionally, and financially draining to be the sandwich generation, having to care for both parents and children at the same time.

PARTICIPATING IN CLINICAL RESEARCH

An enormous number of research studies are going on across the world, mostly aimed at finding better treatments for AD. It is only through these studies that more effective treatments and eventually a cure will be found. Participating in a clinical research study has several key advantages. The screening process can provide the most advanced diagnostic approaches, such as brain scans that can identify amyloid plaques in the brain. The subject will get close monitoring that is typically not available in most medical offices. The experimental treatments may deliver benefits that would otherwise not be possible with present drugs. On a bigger scale, the research studies are the only way to identify novel therapies and perhaps cures for NCDs. Many people dislike research studies and do not want to feel like "guinea pigs." They worry about probable side effects, or about being on a placebo instead of the real medication. These worries are real but must be considered against the possible benefits for both the individual and society.

Chapter 5

Providing Care Through the Middle Stage

It might surprise you that a sizable portion of people with obvious signs of dementia and considerable cognitive impairment do not receive a diagnosis until the disease has progressed to a moderate stage. The reason for this delay in identification is that many people with cognitive decline mistakenly attribute their symptoms to aging and do not consider them serious issues. Others choose not to seek medical attention or visit their primary care physician, never consulting an NCD expert. Delay in diagnosis can lead to a wide range of catastrophes, such as irreversible brain damage, accelerated cognitive and physical decline, harm to oneself or others due to poor decision-making while driving or engaging in other potentially dangerous activities, harm from improper management of medical conditions or medications, financial exploitation, abuse and neglect, family disputes, and legal disputes over wills, to name a few. Once mild stages turn into moderate ones, the window for effective intervention with many different types of NCDs starts to shut quickly.

However, how do we recognize the difference between mild and moderate stages, and why is this crucial? Less insight, more impaired judgment, and more trouble managing activities like driving, cooking, managing finances, and maintaining personal cleanliness are all signs that a person's mental condition is deteriorating into more moderate stages of impairment. These growing impairments result in a significant rise in care requirements as well as an increased risk of unintentional damage to oneself or others. A person repeats questions repeatedly, for example, and there are significant issues managing daily plans and activities, according to caregivers who frequently note that the person's memory lapses and other cognitive deficiencies are more obvious. People with moderately advanced NCDs will score between 10 and 20 on the Mini-Mental State Examination, and rigorous neuropsychological testing will reveal significant cognitive impairment in several different cognitive domains.

Maintaining a Schedule of Daily Activities

While a person with an NCD can still participate in most of the activities they love even into the early stages, this ability alters as the disease progresses. The ability to travel freely, participate in sports and games, manage a hobby, perform volunteer work, and communicate with friends and family as before cognitive impairment sets in is all taken away with the loss of cognitive capacities.

Cognitive decline may be exacerbated by behavioral and mood changes that interfere with daily tasks, such as sadness, anxiety, restlessness, apathy, and anger. Because they are afraid of what to do with the person, family and friends may avoid spending time with them. What, for instance, do a person's poker friends still see them when they are no longer able to play poker? Losing friends, social circles, and hobbies that once provided a lot of support and joy can be tough for caregivers to handle.

At this time, it's crucial to assess the abilities and limitations of the affected person. Make a list of the activities they once enjoyed, and then determine whether they can still perform them fully, partially, or not at all. Exist any adaptations that offer a similar level of enjoyment? Are there any easier card games that someone who used to love playing cards would enjoy if they can't remember enough strategy to play bridge, for instance? Are there day trips that can evoke the same sense of adventure if someone can't travel abroad as easily anymore?

Here are a few general tactics to think about:

- **Build your social portfolio.** Together, make a list of all prospective hobbies and skills, as if you were evaluating the person's assets. What activities does the person enjoy? What holds significance for him or her? Limitations are nothing to worry about just yet. Sort these skills and hobbies into four groups: those that demand a lot of mobility and energy (like playing Bridge) against those that can be done with little mobility and/or energy (like listening to music); those that can be done alone versus those that require a group (watching a movie on television). In his book The Mature Mind, geriatric psychiatrist Gene Cohen explains how the social portfolio concept came to be.

- **Make adjustments.** Review the list of interests as provided, and consider whether ones are still feasible to pursue and any modifications that might be required. Here, use your imagination and perhaps get advice from a person who manages a senior day program. Remember that these modifications are made for the person and not necessarily for you or other family members; as a result, even if an activity is not your first choice, the person with the NCD may love it. Accept it and make an effort to view the situation from that person's perspective.

- **Count on your senses.** The senses take on increased significance as a guide to daily experience when cognitive capacities deteriorate. Consider engaging in sensory-rich activities like listening to music, baking, or visiting gardens. Without respect to memory, the creative arts provide various engaging and profound performances and activities.

- **Involve others.** Participate in these activities with your family, friends, and coworkers. It is frequently because they are unsure of what to do. Those long-time friends seem to avoid caretakers and the person with the NCD. Please provide them with direction and involve them in a planned activity. They'll support it and lend their enthusiasm and ingenuity to it. Children and grandkids are fantastic at participating and don't really care about what the person used to be or could do; they just appreciate the occasion and having a cherished parent or grandparent around.

Here is a list of activities that are ideal for people with moderate stages of NCDs because they stimulate the senses and draw on still-present strengths, are secure and reasonably easy to plan and execute, and can involve family and friends:

- *At-home activities:* Play cards, look through old photo albums or scrapbooks, browse magazines, cook or bake with someone, listen to music or audiobooks, take care of a plant, spend time with a pet, complete simple chores, watch sports, and load an iPod with music the person might enjoy listening to (to learn more about this last suggestion, click here).

- *In the backyard and neighborhood:* Play croquet, visit neighbors, swim, do some basic gardening or yard work, walk around the area, or bring friends or family over for a BBQ.

- *In the neighborhood:* Attend religious services, go to the movies or a restaurant, go to a museum or nature reserve

nearby, visit friends and family, go to a senior center, play
cards, go to a casino, take day trips to nearby attractions,
stroll through a mall, get some ice cream or a snack, or
pick up and deliver a treat for the grandchildren.

All of these tasks appear to be pretty simple and clear, but the
trick is to arrange and streamline them in terms of time, help,
materials, and the time of day. Bring along your relatives and
friends and let them know how they can assist. Keep excursions
brief and schedule them for a time of day when the person with
the NCD will be most active and interested. Do not become
discouraged if the person expresses some resistance, loss of
interest, or apathy. Simply persevere, and eventually, a good
rhythm will emerge. Do not be afraid to enlist the aid of others.
Be their mentor because many friends and family members want
to participate but are unsure how.

There are many different methods to involve kids and grandkids
in activities. So that you can :text, call, and access information,
have them teach you how to network on a computer or mobile
device. To engage and amuse the person with the NCD:

1. Ask them to find some games, videos, or other intriguing
    stuff on an iPad or computer.
2. Allow them to make or cook a traditional family recipe
    with the afflicted individual.
3. Talk about the person's life, family history, and historical
    tales and lessons while you show them antique pictures.
4. Together, recite or sing religious prayers and perform
    rites.

Children require precise, well-defined, and level-appropriate
structured tasks. It is encouraging to observe the impact these
encounters can have on kids.

Adult daycare services that cater to those with mild stages of
NCDs are often available in a variety of alternatives in most

communities. These are sponsored by a wide range of organizations, including senior facilities supported by the city, churches or community centers, charities like Easter Seals, and for-profit companies. Even though many programs are free or inexpensive, others can have high daily fees, particularly if meals and transportation are included. Check to see if the activities are catered to the level of the disabled individual before committing to a program. Allow him or her to test it out for one or two days to determine if it's a good fit. Even if there is a fee, it may be less expensive than hiring an assistant for those same hours. For people who would otherwise stay at home alone and bored, the sociability and structure of the activities can be quite helpful.

Increasing Care Needs

The most significant impact on caregivers during the mild stages of NCDs may be rising care needs. These requirements increase in line with the areas of cognitive impairment, such as forgetting appointments and other daily events (memory problems), having trouble understanding instructions or expressing thoughts or concerns (language impairment or aphasia), not being able to recognize familiar people, places, or things (recognition impairment or agnosia, and visuospatial impairment), forgetting how to perform basic and complex tasks (apraxia), and having trouble organizing and prioritizing tasks (executive dysfunction). Here, we'll go over a few important care requirements.

Supervision

Over time, the amount of supervision needed to maintain the patient's safety throughout the moderate stages of sickness will rise, eventually necessitating 24-hour surveillance. Take into account the following inquiries as you determine the level of supervision. What are the risks to the person if they are left alone:

- Wandering off and becoming disoriented?

- Falling or becoming hurt and being unsure on how to get assistance?
- Forgetting to put out a fire on the stove? Leaving the water running and causing a flood?
- Allowing a stranger into your home?
- Are you handling a medical emergency?

In each of these scenarios, a person's capacity to stay safe depends on their ability to avoid or anticipate risky situations, to recognize when a threat exists, and to be able to get assistance by looking for a neighbor or dialing 911. All of these essential cognitive domains inevitably deteriorate in the middle stages of NCDs. The only method to ensure maximum safety is to have someone on duty constantly, either living there or staying nearby and conducting frequent check-ins.

Individuals with moderate disability frequently do not receive this monitoring owing to a lack of social or financial means, a lack of awareness of the hazards, or an aversion to receiving assistance. Caretakers may occasionally exaggerate the patient's mental capacity or assume that nothing will happen in the future because nothing has happened so far. This strategy is possibly careless and dangerous. The following are a few options for enhancing supervision:

- Arrange for the person to live with a relative.
- Employ assistants or companions to stay with them.
- Place the person in a nursing home or assisted living facility.

Neighbors are frequently asked to provide supervision in smaller or more tight-knit communities, but this is not a reliable solution and depends on these people's skills, tolerance, and goodwill. Additionally, it invites potential abuse. It is crucial that if family members are asked to assist, they truly have the time, inclination, incentive, and capacity to do so. Older spouses occasionally have cognitive or physical limits when it comes to assisting with hygiene problems or agitation.

HYGIENE

For a variety of reasons, hygiene can become a problem during the moderate stages, and it frequently presents the most distressing and challenging challenges for caregivers. Many people with impairments start to lose track of when and how to groom themselves properly, and occasionally they even refuse to take regular showers or change their clothes. This is brought on by a loss of perspective, lack of interest in or comprehension of the value of social graces, and a decreased capacity to maintain personal hygiene and grooming. Additionally, as the NCD worsens, the likelihood of bowel and urinary incontinence rises, increasing the risk of accidents. The person with the impairment might not be as aware of urges to use the restroom or be unable to get together quickly enough to get there. Accidents can be embarrassing for the individual who experiences them as well as for the caregiver, mainly if the individual does not realize what has occurred, tries to hide it, or objects to have cleaned up. Accidents can cause people to avoid social situations. Here are a few fundamental methods for handling hygiene issues:

Create a Routine:

According to the person's prior grooming habits, set aside specific morning and evening times, locations, and days for grooming. Establish regular bathroom breaks for the person throughout the day if they experience frequent bladder and bowel incontinence. Establish a routine for visiting the hairdresser and manicurist so that you may maintain excellent grooming while making the experience pleasurable and respectable.

Have Respect for Privacy and Dignity:

Reluctance to accept help is frequently caused by a person's reluctance to allow others to assist them with very private and perhaps embarrassing actions. This could be the reason the individual chooses to stroll around in soiled underwear rather than let a family member see them undressed or assist them in cleaning up. To maintain privacy and dignity, caregivers should practice good hygiene.

Provide Cues:

The individual will require prompts, visual cues, supervision, and, if necessary, hands-on assistance to choose and put on clothing, clean up, and maintain a presentable appearance. As a person advances into later moderate and severe stages and finds it harder and harder to actually use a toothbrush, comb, razor, and other basic grooming tools, hands-on care becomes even more important.

Rule Out Medical Conditions:

Medical conditions or drugs, such as tooth decay and infections, excessive scratching or rubbing on skin, constipation, infections, and many other causes, might be associated with hygiene problems such as mouth or body odors, rashes, and incontinence. Always have your primary care doctor and other specialists (dentists, podiatrists, dermatologists) assess your symptoms and recommend the best course of action.

Be Ready:

Always have enough grooming and incontinence supplies on-hand, such as rubber or plastic gloves, hand sanitizer, hygienic wipes, protective underwear, and a change of clothes.

As NCDs worsen, maintaining good hygiene can be difficult, but it is crucial for maintaining health as well as comfort, confidence, and dignity. Many people still feel good when they feel and look clean and well-groomed, even in the later stages of sickness.

Security for the Person and the Home:

People with moderately advanced NCDs are typically still mobile and motivated to move around and keep busy. While this energy can be used to carry out daily tasks, it can also make them more challenging and even dangerous because the person cannot move around safely, operate appliances safely, and get help if needed. 24-hour monitoring is required as patients enter their illnesses' late-moderate and severe phases. In the absence of that, the individual and their home environment need to be protected and made as comfortable as possible. Some of the following may fall under this:

Prepare and Provide Forms of Identification:

The impaired person needs to have an identification bracelet and wallet card made so that if they get lost and wander outside the house, someone will know who they are and who to call. The MedicAlert® + Alzheimer's Association Safe Return® program, developed by the Alzheimer's Association, offers missing people with NCDs a 24-hour emergency response. To provide GPS tracking for people with dementia, the Alzheimer's Association also offers improved systems named Comfort Zone® and Comfort Zone Check-In®.

Safe Exits:

Have secure locks on the doors and bells that sound when the door is opened if the person has a tendency to wander and has trouble recognizing familiar places to stop them from leaving unnoticed or unaided. Sometimes a simple fix for frequent exits is a chain link on the entrance that is out of sight. Near pools, it's crucial to have secure exits.

Clear the Clutter:

Moving around in a tidy, orderly, and minimally furnished home is simpler and safer. Look for potential dangers and obstacles as you walk around the house, such as hanging rugs, electrical cords that are in the way, sharp corners, and unnoticed steps.

Label and Maintain Stability:

- Put labels or photos on the doors, cabinets, drawers, and containers that the person will need to open to get at things like clothing, socks, toothpaste, dining utensils, glasses, and bowls. To help them remember where you put your shoes, wallet, keys, and other regularly used goods, designate stable spots for them and mark them. This may lessen the frustration associated with having trouble locating things.

- Create lengthy lists. Make extensive lists of frequently used phone numbers, family and friends, and significant dates (with photos, if appropriate) to create an external memory of people, important numbers, and events. Consider keeping these lists in a visible location in a colorful, clearly labeled binder. A large calendar with a list of all upcoming events and days crossed off on it should be placed in a prominent, stable location to help with orientation.

- Inspect the knobs and switches. Consider whether there is a chance that the stove, water faucets, or other appliances will be left on and not properly monitored if the individual lives alone or is left alone for a portion of the day. Examine each switch and knob on these things to see if there's any way to make it safer, less convenient, or inactive. Even when a companion is there, a person can get up in the middle of the night, take a bath or boil water for tea, and end up starting a fire, flooding the house, getting burned, or falling into a tub of water.

This process of protecting the person and home indeed necessitates visualizing numerous disasters. Still, it is better to spend some time thinking about and averting these scenarios than to ignore them and assume nothing will happen. Sadly, horrible things can occur when there is insufficient planning and oversight.

Identifying Possible Risks:

Individuals can no longer operate vehicles, power tools, and weapons with the same level of skill and safety awareness due to the cognitive changes brought on by moderate stages of NCDs. They may disregard safety regulations like signaling appropriately or paying attention to road signs while driving, wearing safety goggles while using an electric saw or other power tools, or waiting to fire a rifle before checking for other hunters due to decreased insight and judgment, frontal lobe impairment, and impaired visuospatial skills. The most frequent worry is driving, mainly if someone depends on it to shop and run errands, if their partner doesn't drive, or if they have no transportation. Because driving restrictions are strongly associated with losing independence, many impaired people fight them. Keep in mind that research clearly shows that driving with a moderate stage NCD is as risky as driving drunk. An increase in minor collisions, tickets for moving violations, and regular disregard for traffic laws are all indications that the person shouldn't be driving. Although giving up these activities is challenging, a growing impairment necessitates it. Here are some suggestions:

- In the very early to intermediate stages, driving, use of power tools, or use of firearms for hunting should be closely supervised during the day and only when the person is fully attentive and compliant with instructions.

- All of these activities must be disallowed after the early to intermediate stages or when risky behaviors have already been shown, and access to car keys, power tools, and weapons must be constrained.

- It's crucial to arrange dependable and convenient alternate transportation for social activities, doctor's appointments, and shopping.

- To evaluate a driver's ability, memory centers provide computerized and on-road driving exams.

- Given the expected progression of the condition, the American Academy of Neurology advises that drivers with early-stage dementia undertake on-road testing again and routine reassessment every six months at the very least.

None of these activities can be permitted by the late to moderate stages due to the high risk of serious harm or even death. Even if being proactive results in mental distress, it is preferable to risk suffering a catastrophic accident, losing property, and probable legal repercussions.

Management of Finances:

Along with waning insight, judgment, mathematical abilities, and executive function is the ability to balance a checkbook and make well-reasoned decisions about handling finances. Sadly, some criminals prey on cognitively impaired individuals who do not have built-in safeguards to prevent financial exploitation and inevitable ruin. These safeguards include the following:

- Have clear documentation of the NCD in a medical record. Without this documentation, the authorities have little ground to go after criminals who financially exploit the cognitively impaired person.

- Make an inventory of cash, valuables, and checkbooks and keep them in safe, locked locations with access restricted to designated caregivers, attorneys, or accountants who are helping to manage finances.

- Complete well-documented estate planning before significant cognitive impairment. Before signing any legal contracts, the person should have a neuropsychological evaluation to ascertain whether they can make a financial decision.

- Take into account routing all mail and phone calls to a single individual who can examine all inquiries. As a result, criminals won't be able to approach the intoxicated person directly.

Having an NCD, even in the intermediate stages, does not mean that a person cannot engage in financial decisions. Still, it does suggest the need for assistance and precise documentation. More straightforward steps can be used to make complex decisions, and it is still possible to express preferences and use them as guidelines, such as by giving others modest-sized gifts. The appointment of surrogate decision-makers can protect the process, but these people must be dependable, understand the impaired person's intentions, and act in the person's best interests.

Chapter 6

Advanced Stages of Caregiving

Neurocognitive disorders do not always proceed to more severe phases. Caregiving techniques for mild to moderate levels of impairment can be used throughout the entire course of vascular dementias and NCDs caused by medical conditions because they frequently remain constant or only slightly worsen. However, with progressive NCDs like frontotemporal dementia, dementia with Lewy bodies, Alzheimer's disease, and others; a person's condition will unavoidably deteriorate over years until they are entirely dependent on others for help with most, if not all, of their daily activities. In this severe stage of sickness, care requirements significantly increase, necessitating more support from people with specialized training. Without such assistance, even the best caretaker may become overwhelmed.

At this point, the main goal of the caregiver is to provide for the severely disabled person's fundamental needs in terms of nourishment, hydration, hygiene, sleep, regulation of physical and mental pain and discomfort, and basic affection and sensory stimulation. Going above and beyond these criteria frequently results in time, money, and energy waste and is ultimately futile. Giving someone with AD and severe aphasia pricey speech therapy is one illustration. The therapy will result in negligible gains that swiftly disappear without any discernible benefit, but it will cost money and cause the affected individual frustration. The use of music therapy to stimulate verbal abilities through song or prayer would be a preferable approach, as will be discussed.

In general, if one or more of the following conditions exist, a person may be thought to be in advanced stages of an NCD:

- Even with mobility aids, the person is unable to walk or move around.
- In the event of a crisis, the individual is unable to leave the situation.
- In an emergency, the person is unable to call for assistance.
- The person can no longer effectively communicate vocally.
- The individual is lost in terms of time, location, and people.
- The affected person is unable to eat, clothe, or clean themselves.
- Both bladder and bowel control is gone.
- The subject receives a Mini-Mental State Examination score of 10 or less.

Of course, there are other indicators as well, and speaking with the treating doctor is crucial to determining the sickness stage and the overall care requirements.

Gems for Understanding Neurological Disorder

Trying to fathom what someone with significant cognitive impairment is thinking and feeling can be one of the biggest obstacles to comprehending them. Their speech is frequently muddled or absurd, and it can be challenging to understand how they move and behave. The nationally renowned occupational therapist and NCD expert, Teepa Snow, created one of the best and most compassionate guides with her book, Dementia Caregiver Guide. Snow offers a beautiful, insightful, and encouraging framework for comprehending people with NCDs called the Teepa Show.

Her levels are unique from every other staging in that they are approachable for both caretakers and professionals and place an equal emphasis on strengths that are still there as well as weaknesses. As Snow notes in her book, these levels are not entirely defined and can alter over time depending on the context and work; as a result, a person may exhibit traits from numerous levels. The levels serve as "indicators" of a person's inner experiences and talents rather than as judgmental labels. These levels favor the individual over the illness, as seen by the fact that they are named after jewels. The following is a summary of these levels:

Ruby: Severe brain dysfunction. The person can make large motions, but their fine motor abilities are deteriorating. The person can duplicate instructions but not understand them, and they struggle to adapt to change. The individual can still react appropriately to rhythmic activities involving sensory input, such as music and movement. The daily schedule must be planned while remaining adaptable to the individual's sleep-wake cycle. Due to their limited mobility, some activities may require two caretakers.

Diamond: Subtle cognitive alterations. The individual does best when given structure, yet they can still excel.

Emerald: Mild cognitive alterations. Despite errors, mishaps, communication difficulties, and a lack of complete awareness of their deficiencies, the person functions but is no longer independent.

Amber: Mild to serious cognitive impairment. The individual is present and concentrates on the senses. "Exploration without safety knowledge" exists. Delaying gratification is not always possible. The person requires structure, direction, and visual cues from caregivers before verbal ones, along with regular breaks to prevent overstimulation and irritation.

Sapphire: Aging normally without an NCD. Age-related difficulties exist and require work to overcome, but learning is attainable.

Pearl: Advanced NCD. Although there are levels of ability that still provide connection, there is a loss of mobility and a restricted ability to engage with the outer world. Care requires nonverbal messages. The surroundings should be relaxing and stimulating to the senses.

The fundamental benefit of Teepa Snow's constructive strategy is the practical advice she offers for caring for patients who are suffering from severe sickness when many carers experience stress or confusion. Snow has produced some beneficial videos that offer incredibly sensible and practical techniques of communicating with people who have disabilities.

The connection between the caregiver and the person with the NCD, which varies substantially in advanced stages of sickness, can also be managed with the use of the Gems. By necessity, the caregiver must take on a greater parental role. Verbal communication frequently breaks down, and the caregiver no longer experiences nearly as much of the shared satisfaction that they used to with the affected person. The ability of a spouse to seek advice on domestic, monetary, or familial issues, as well as physical or sexual contact, shall be prohibited. Children and grandchildren who can no longer interact with the person in the way they did previously will be unable to access family history and anecdotes.

During these stages, the sense of loss that caregivers and loved ones experience is heightened, and emotions such as sadness, melancholy, anger, resentment, loneliness, and even despair may intensify. However, although the relationship has changed, it is still present, and occasionally, there may be deeper connections than before.

Supervision

Due to their level of confusion and disorientation and the resulting risk of injury or emotional distress, people with severe stage NCDs cannot be left unattended. Cleanliness, orderliness, accessibility, security, and accessibility of both persons and supplies for all care requirements are required in the setting. Many caregivers choose long-term care at this point because they can no longer keep the person they are caring for at home. It is feasible to keep someone at home as long as there is sufficient monitoring and care, especially for those who are unable to walk or speak. Never leave someone in such a state alone at home; doing so puts them at risk for serious harm and may even land them in legal trouble if the police or other protective services are called to the scene. Remember that it takes more than just being present to help; it also takes someone who can comprehend the person's situation and react correctly. The chances of subpar care and even damage are therefore increased when a youngster or an inexperienced neighbor is asked to maintain watch.

Is therapy still required?

Whether cognitive-function-improving drugs or other NCD treatments are still worthwhile throughout advanced stages of sickness is a subject that caregivers frequently ask. These treatments are obviously not going to cure the condition, and the advantages are at most minor. This is a judgment call that must be based on the treatment's objectives and if specified in advance in advance directives, the wishes of the impaired person. However, there are a few things to remember.

Why upset the balance? Even though it may take some time for acetylcholinesterase inhibitors or memantine to have a noticeable effect, research results have shown some benefit from ongoing use (or even starting) of these medications. When these medications are stopped, in some situations, there is a rapid loss in function that can be challenging, if not impossible, to restore. Consider the possible repercussions of quitting a medicine whose advantages exist but are not always obvious if the patient is generally stable.

- Pay attention to hardship and agony. There are numerous drugs that can be used to treat uncomfortable or painful conditions when they are at their worst, including those for skin rashes and itching, nasal and bronchial congestion, joint discomfort, insomnia, headache, and other things. Without using extensive medical treatments, many problems can be resolved.

- Is there room for further development? Mood, behavior, sleep, and hunger issues can always be resolved, regardless of the kind of NCD, even in the most advanced stages of the condition. Sometimes treating one or more of these related issues might enhance mental function and cognition as well.

Remaining Engaged in Positive and Energizing Activities

For someone with significant cognitive impairment, finding pleasurable, fulfilling, and stimulating hobbies is, in some respects, less difficult than with earlier stages. Activities must be highly controlled, portable, and mostly centered on sensory engagement because people have reduced ability to participate vocally and physically. Caretakers and others must offer the framework and external incentive since people who have diminished mobility, disorientation, apathy, and impaired executive function are unable to come up with their own ideas or motivate themselves. Focus on sensory activities that the person has previously enjoyed, but don't keep them there. Encourage family members, especially the younger ones, to participate in the activity. Do not worry if the activity looks too juvenile or "below" the person; instead, consider it from his or her perspective. If the person does not want to or is not enjoying the activity, do not make them participate. The following is a list of possible activities:

Arousal of the Senses

- Prepare and sample unique dishes, such as baked goods.
- Identify various spices by smell.
- Fill pots with flowers.
- Go to a beautiful park or garden; stroll along a beach boardwalk at dusk.
- Use fragrant lotions to massage your hands.
- Massage your back, arms, or hands gently.
- Take in musical or instrumental performances.
- Go to a museum to view the art.

Stimulation of Memory

- Examine recent or vintage photos and pinpoint the individuals or locations.
- Take in your favorite or well-known musical selections.
- Go over any lingering recollections of early encounters.
- Pay a visit to enduring friends or relations.
- Interact in a first language that you both still know.

Activities between Generations

- Request that they tell a younger person about their past.
- Enlist the assistance of younger family members in decorating the person's space, wheelchair, or walker.
- Engage in easy joint arts & crafts projects.
- Make and sample a recipe from the family.
- Listen to music together or watch a movie.

- Plant something that will grow, always reminding youngsters of the visit.

Physical Exercise

- Participate in chair yoga, light stretching, or other exercises.
- Engage in simple games like horseshoe throwing, catching and tossing a ball, lounging on a pier, and fishing.
- Go for a stroll through the neighborhood or a nearby park.
- Carry out easy domestic tasks together.

Religious, Spiritual and Cultural Activities

- Participate in a religious event.
- Sing or read prayers aloud together.
- Seek out clerics.
- Sing or listen to religious or folk music.
- Share in rituals and holiday celebrations.

Keep in mind that with all of these activities, you can still access memories and abilities that are still there, such as the ability to speak a language you learned as a child, say prayers, partake in long-standing rituals, sing, or dance. Up until the very last stages of the disease, the senses are still functional and allow for interaction with the outside world.

Life-Ending Problems

Every progressive NCD eventually leads to a stage where the affected person loses all fundamental abilities, including the capacity to walk, talk, and eventually swallow. Bedridden people run the risk of developing decubitus ulcers, which are sores that break the skin. Lack of speech makes it difficult for a person to express wants or distress; these are instead shown by writhing, agitation, or shouting. The danger of dehydration and malnutrition increases when swallowing is impaired because it causes loss of food and liquid intake. Additionally, it raises the chance that food fragments will inhale and cause aspiration pneumonia in the lungs. At this time, the person typically has a few months to live, with infections, dehydration, or untreated medical conditions frequently being the cause of death. Because medical care can extend a person's life despite significant impairment, end-of-life issues frequently occur at this time. At this point, caregivers want to avoid pain and suffering, but many wonder if it is worthwhile to delay death when the quality of life is so poor.

End Stage Treatment Decisions

It is not necessary to maintain them at the final, terminal stage because there is no discernible benefit. What about the management of medical conditions? Advance directives are crucial in this situation because they outline the handicapped person's preferences. It is ideal if the individual has stated in writing what kind of treatment they desire to receive when they are unable to make decisions for themselves, including whether to undergo resuscitation in the event of cardiac arrest or breathing cessation. All long-term care facilities demand that families either present a pre-existing document or decide if they want the patient to be revived at the time of admission. At this point, a "do not resuscitate" (DNR) order is justified because there is little possibility the patient will recover from cardiac arrest.

However, caregivers must be aware that DNR orders only apply to emergency resuscitation (in which case medical personnel administer chest compressions and insert a breathing tube in the patient's throat), and that a DNR order does *not* preclude the doctor from performing ordinary medical procedures. The level to which the caregivers desire to provide this care must be discussed with the physician.

The most typical strategy in treating end-stage NCDs is to treat minor issues including coughs, minor scrapes or wounds, constipation, diarrhea, and skin itching that would otherwise result in excessive pain or discomfort. However, what if the patient has pneumonia? Would they provide antibiotics intravenously? additional oxygen? Painkillers? Referral to a hospice program is suitable if the intention is to offer comfort or palliative treatment. In that case, the hospice staff will maintain the patient's comfort without actively treating the underlying sickness. The emotional responses to such circumstances might make decision-making more difficult, even with explicit directives.

Tube Feeding Pros and Cons

When a person experiences difficulty swallowing, they run the risk of choking on food and aspirating it into their lungs, where it might infect them. Traditionally, oral feeding was kept up for as long as feasible and occasionally supplemented with fluids or nutritional supplements given by an intravenous tube or feeding tube temporarily inserted in the stomach through the nose. However, since the 1980s, medical professionals have been able to permanently implant a percutaneous gastrostomy, or PEG tube, through the abdominal wall and into the stomach to deliver routine nutritional infusions. This tube feeding can offer many people a lifeline during their rehabilitation from a stroke or similar condition that prevents them from eating. However, it's unclear whether tube feeding actually enhances the quality of life or lengthens survival for those with end-stage NCDs. It may result in nausea, vomiting, bloating, stomach pain, infections at the tube site, and nausea and/or vomiting. Before making a final choice, caregivers must carefully consider all of these advantages and disadvantages in a discussion with the patient's physician and surgeon.

Brain Donation

Some people express a desire to donate their brains to science after passing away; sometimes organizations ask caretakers and relatives to donate the brain of the afflicted person. Either way, there are brain banks in several major cities that welcome these donations since it enables them to understand different NCDs in greater detail.

Families receive a thorough report that details the precise pathology in the brain, which in turn identifies the precise type of NCD the person had, in addition to contributing to the advancement of scientific research. Families may find this information useful in recognizing their risk factors on occasion. Numerous causes of cognitive impairment are revealed in the reports in many situations, differing from the clinical assessments made before the patient passed away.

To find out the precise steps for brain donation, potential donors can get in touch with a local brain bank. It is advisable to make plans before passing away and to make sure that everyone in the family is on board. A funeral and burial are not prevented by brain donation, and they are frequently not even postponed. Major hospitals and medical facilities frequently house brain banks. Once someone has passed away, they will rapidly remove the brain (some institutions also offer the option to perform a full autopsy), then transfer the body to a chosen funeral home. Donating a brain is free of charge.

Chapter 7

The Caregiver

One might assume that the physical and financial strain of caring for loved ones with dementia would be enough to wear anyone out or that these issues would be the biggest challenge. However, until you are actually in this situation, you won't realize how much more difficult it is on an emotional and mental level as a result of witnessing your parents in this situation.

No one will ever question how painful it is to witness loved ones in discomfort, suffering, or struggling with chores they formerly took for granted. Both the elderly and those who care for them find the aging process challenging. You need to retain your composure in this scenario and do your best to maintain your parents' quality of life while keeping your own mental and physical needs in mind. The caregiver also needs to be taken care of; if you don't take care of yourself first, who will take care of your parents?

Learn:

If your loved one has a condition that could be causing him more problems or hastening his decline, his aging process may be altered and cannot be explained by the aging process alone. By knowing as much as you can about the specific illness or condition that may be preventing him, try to understand him better.

Support:

You are your loved one's bulwark; you keep him active and serve as his primary source of sustenance. You'll need the same kind of support throughout this period, so talk to your partner, your grown children, and your siblings and ask for help or guidance. If everything else fails, you can vent in one of the available caregiver support groups. Ask about support groups when you call your neighborhood community center.

Optimism:

There isn't much you can do to stop your loved one's illness from worsening; all you can do is try to make things easier for them. And what better way to make things easier than by maintaining your optimism? You and your loved one are related, after all; lighten the mood by telling a secret joke, going out to dine, or recalling earlier times.

Diversion:

Anything is preferable to leaning into negativity if you can't keep things on a positive note. Distract them with anything you can think of if you sense the conversation is going on a wrong path or if your loved one has started to become visibly quiet with their thoughts. How is the weather right now? Anything to divert attention from the inevitable though (now) avoidable or inquire about an antique picture frame that might be sitting nearby.

Exercise:

Exercise has been shown to reduce stress and fight depression, both of which are prevalent in the elderly. If your loved one is still mobile, you should do all your power to retain it and make sure they are as mobile as possible by engaging in physical activity, stretching, or walking. Exercise is beneficial for you as well, and you can exercise together. Workout is:

1. Beneficial for your mental and physical wellness.

2. A task that involves several people.
3. The opportunity to go outside and breathe fresh air.

Planning:

The earlier you start planning, the sooner your loved one may be able to get it out of their thoughts as well. This is because it is best done when your loved one is still mentally stable. Get your papers, such as the will and a power of attorney, out of the way by hiring an elder care lawyer. The DNR (do not resuscitate) option and potential life support should also be considered and discussed with your loved one.

Meaningful Activities:

Meaningful activities are always good for getting the blood flowing and returning the reason we carry on with life. Making a photo collage or even looking through old photo albums might be helpful. If your loved one enjoys music, you might also consider taking them to the theatre. Go to a museum, and feed the ducks in the park—anything to rekindle the tiniest spark.

Rest:

Always take breaks, and I don't just mean a 10-minute peaceful sit-down in the living room. If you are the sole caretaker for a loved one, consider occasionally hiring an aide so you may take a break and realize that you have a life of your own. If you have siblings willing to help out occasionally, give them specific instructions on what needs to be done, such as taking medication, and set aside time for them to come so you can take a well-earned break.

Respect:

It might be more straightforward for respect to erode when your parent starts to rely more and more on you. Keep in mind that he is still your parent and cannot change the way he is. If he can still make decisions, respect him and his choices. Instead of giving orders, seek his input on care strategies or routine modifications. This is still his life, and he should hold on to it and all the decisions that come with it for as long as he can. You may be managing his health and well-being.

Kindness:

The elderly often have shorter fuses, which can make things more challenging regarding things like eating, medication, and occasionally even hygiene. This will be even harder if your loved one has bad habits like drinking or smoking that he can't or doesn't want to give up. He may be elderly and conscious of the end of his life, so he likely doesn't see anything wrong with what he is doing right now. You may know what is best for him and what needs to be done and avoided to prolong his health. The process of enforcing what has to be done will go more smoothly if you choose your words carefully and act with kindness.

Dignity:

If you aren't the one losing your dignity, it can be not easy to notice. Put yourself in your loved ones' position and do your best to imagine what that could be like to help you develop empathy. Some apparent measures to maintain dignity include showering in privacy and keeping up with personal hygiene. Still, some less apparent considerations must be made. Before you go out to dinner, are the clothes on your loved ones clean? He could feel less proud of himself if he appeared and felt unclean. When your siblings come to see you, they will inevitably ask how your parents are doing, and you will inevitably answer them. Is your father present? Hear you, can he? Speaking absentmindedly, significantly when discussing private matters like incontinence, can damage one's dignity.

Reassure the person you care about that aging is a natural process and that there is nothing to be ashamed of. If it helps, you could pay an assistant to take care of your hygiene, so you don't have to. Your parent might object, but you might not.

Individualized Care:

Person-centered care is one of those things that is so clear and right in front of you that you fail to notice it. Although some medical professionals and caregivers have practiced person-centered care in the past, it has only recently emerged as a legitimate method of providing and delivering care.

Person-centered care considers individual differences and how they view treatment, care, medicine, activities, and other variables that affect their general health and welfare. With the advent of person-centered care, medical professionals and you as a caregiver should be aware that patients should be met, spoken to, and dealt with based on their unique personalities and preferences rather than being labeled by their condition. Many health professionals are taught how to approach patients based on their illness or condition and are sometimes even taught lines to say.

Recognize that not everyone wants to be treated in the same conventional manner even though they have the same ailment or condition. While some people prefer constant affirmation and attention, others can prefer solitude. Knowing your loved one's preferences and the methods required to keep or enhance the care he receives is a crucial component of being a good caretaker.

Managing Dementia and Alzheimer's:

Your loved one's condition can deteriorate more quickly if they have Alzheimer's or dementia than if they were aging naturally. From a medical perspective, Alzheimer's and dementia are already challenging conditions to manage; nevertheless, witnessing your parent struggle with one of these crippling diseases can be incredibly distressing as a caregiver.

It is terrible and challenging to see your mother, who gave you life and reared you, gradually lose all memory of who you and your siblings are. As a caregiver, this will have an emotional and mental impact on you that you will carry with you for a very long time, if not forever. Keep in mind that a person is more than simply their recollection. Your parents are still the same person, regardless of what led to this ailment or where it may be in its progression. She might not remember things, but her touch, smile, and voice will all still be the same, and in the end, she will always be the person you love.

Chapter 8

Legal Issues

In the early stages of a neurocognitive disorder, caregivers must consider significant legal considerations. These problems are caused by how NCD symptoms gradually but progressively erode an individual's capacity for independent decision-making and functioning. A thorough neurocognitive evaluation is the best resource for dealing with these problems because it gives essential details about the kind and severity of cognitive impairment that will affect decision-making. Most disagreements over wills, financial gifts, medical expenses, and other crucial decisions arise when there are doubts about the decision-making capacity of the person with the NCD.

Decision Making

When a person has moderate to severe cognitive impairment, caregivers frequently need to step in and assist them in making decisions. The choice could be as straightforward as what to eat for lunch or as complex as whether they require nursing home care. The stakes are higher, and several family members or other parties may have different viewpoints, making medical, financial, and estate planning decisions more difficult. Can someone with moderate Alzheimer's disease (AD) change their will to leave one child out, for instance? Is it possible for someone with a severe NCD to give money to a church? Can those same people choose not to receive cancer chemotherapy? Or give the house's deed to one child but not the other? And what if the primary caregiver of one child wants to make a choice that the other children disagree with? These problems crop up frequently and call for a knowledge of decision-making capacity.

The term "capacity" describes a person's cognitive capability to comprehend and reason about a subject to reach appropriate and sane conclusions. A person's competence to make specific decisions is usually assessed through an interview with a mental health professional, such as a psychologist or psychiatrist. Because the subject can then be questioned about matters pertinent to the inquiry, the examination should evaluate decision-making unique to specific issues, such as whether the person can vote, sign a document, engage in litigation, choose where to reside, and so forth.

Generally speaking, a person who is capable of making judgments should be able to demonstrate that they are aware of the situation, the alternatives available, their specifics, and the outcomes of each. Additionally, the individual must be able to analyze the relevant problems and then clearly articulate a preference. For instance, if someone is asked to decide whether to consent to a medical procedure, they should be able to explain what the procedure entails, the options available to them, and the potential outcomes of each option before weighing their options and communicating their decision to you at various points. Unfortunately, people with NCDs are frequently allowed to make decisions (or are covertly or openly forced to do so) without verifying their actual capacity.

How does capacity testing work? In addition to having a conversation with the patient about their problems, the clinician should do a cognitive screen (as detailed in chapter 2) to evaluate the patient's memory, language, attention, concentration, knowledge, and executive function. [1] An individual's cognitive status can be determined with precision using neuropsychological testing. Someone does not necessarily lack capacity just because they have an NCD. It may imply that they are limited in some ways, but this does not preclude them from exercising good judgment, especially concerning matters with which they have extensive knowledge and expertise. Once more, the disabled individual needs to be evaluated for the current problem. Even people with profound memory loss can communicate their logical choices for what to wear, eat, and do. However, more significant choices might be challenging when dementia is advanced since the repercussions are higher, and the person is less able to express the same choice over time. There are legal procedures to set up substitute decision-makers during these phases, as will be discussed.

One of the most contentious areas of decision-making, when a person has an NCD is the ability to form a will to divide one's property after death. Testamentary capacity is defined as the capability to do so. To have testamentary capability, a person must be aware of their assets, the recipients of their assets (such as the number and names of their spouse and children), and how they desire to be distributed. Wills are typically drafted before someone is diagnosed with an NCD, but issues might occur if there is no will or if it is out of date at the time the person begins to lose cognitive function. There is occasionally concern about undue influence, which occurs when a caregiver or another person dependent on the cognitively impaired person uses persuasion, intimidation, or even threats to persuade them to make decisions that are in their best interests rather than their other potential beneficiaries.

Durable Power of Attorney

The durable power of attorney (DPOA) is a legal arrangement in which a designated person or "agent" is permitted to carry out specific financial and legal transactions on behalf of a person or "principal." That authority will continue (as it is "durable") if the principal becomes incapable due to an NCD or another reason. The DPOA is effective as soon as it is signed; therefore, there is no need for a formal court case to establish the principal's incapacity, and the agent can start carrying out the duties at any time. [2] The decisions the assigned person can make, whether they can use any cash for themselves, and if they are paid for their work are outlined in the DPOA agreements. Sometimes caregivers act as the DPOA, while a family lawyer or accountant may also be chosen. The DPOA offers essential financial protection to persons who might not otherwise be able to handle their finances or might be at risk of having their money taken advantage of without their knowledge. They also offer a quicker and more affordable substitute for applying for guardianship.

Governance and Competency

Competency is a legal term that describes a person's capacity for making wise decisions. The only person who can decide if someone lacks mental competency (is "incompetent" to make decisions, for example) is a judge in a formal court process. Although the phrases capacity and competency are sometimes used interchangeably, it is essential to know the difference between them legally. A person must first undergo an evaluation by one or more (often three) court-appointed examiners who concur that the individual lacks decision-making capacity in one or more of the following categories before being eligible for legal guardianship:

- Choices regarding health care (Examples: deciding whether to get a surgery done, participating in the research)
- Monetary or estate choices (examples: managing property, investment decisions, giving gifts of money, executing a will)

- The home (examples: where to live, with whom, and with what help)
- Civic and legal obligations (examples: voting, marrying, serving on a jury, entering into a contract, participating in legal proceedings, suing or being sued, standing trial or testifying at one)

A judge will evaluate the examiners' conclusions when the examinations are finished, consult with the subject, hear from the counsel on both sides, and then decide. The judge will appoint a guardian, conservator, or fiduciary (depending on the word used in that country) to make decisions on behalf of the incompetent individual if they are judged to be incapable. The guardianship may also be subject to limitations set down by the judge, some privileges being granted but not others. The guardian is then permitted to function as the incapacitated person's surrogate and make choices. Guardians cannot go against the person's best interests and have some legal obligations and restrictions.

Unless otherwise demonstrated, people are considered to be competent for legal purposes. Therefore, the person contesting a person's capacity for decision-making has the burden of proof. The judge and the selected examiners will decide whether or not a person's decisions are sound; you cannot infer this from the fact that they have an NCD. Remember that even those with intact decision-making abilities occasionally behave erratically and are reluctant to assist.

When ought you to think about requesting guardianship? Technically, even though they lack legal authority, most carers serve as de facto guardians for people with moderate to severe impairments. This informal setting works well as long as the individual or others don't question the caregiver's judgments. For instance, if a wife took her moderately cognitively impaired husband to a lawyer to have a new will created and signed, and the impaired person was able to participate, agree, and sign for the changes, there would be no issues unless someone with a stake in the will, such as a son or daughter, contested the person's capacity to make legal decisions. Given the repercussions, having guardianship would prevent the disabled person from changing a will rather than allowing the guardian to do so. In other words, guardianship is more about preventing the impaired person from making poor judgments that could result in self-harm or cause them to be exploited, abused, or impoverished than empowering the guardian.

Undoubtedly, a more widespread but costly method of assuming responsibility for someone with an NCD is legal guardianship. However, there are significant restrictions even with guardianship. For instance, in most states, a legal guardian cannot sign a patient into a mental health facility; instead, the patient must be placed in a temporary legal status that a judge must finally approve. As a result, creating a DPOA is more accessible, cheaper, and will generally achieve the same objectives.

Prior Directives

Some of the most significant and heavy decisions we make in life are prompted by medical and end-of-life issues, but many people with NCDs are unable to engage in them reasonably. Advance directives are meant to lay out a person's desires in advance regarding these matters and designate a surrogate or proxy to act on their behalf and make decisions when the individual cannot. Advance directives are a collection of legal documents that a person drafts and signs before losing mental capacity. They may include the following:

- A proxy directive appoints a surrogate to act on behalf of the person deciding the case of mental impairment. The surrogate may be named as a health care proxy or a durable power of attorney for health care. The most typical proxies chosen are spouses and adult children.

- A living will that outlines a person's intentions for medical
  decisions when they cannot make them for themselves.

All healthcare companies must tell all patients about advance
directives since the Patient Self-Determination Act was passed in
1990.

Advance directives are therefore meant for everyone and are not
just utilized in the case of NCDs. A lawyer can provide you with
relevant documentation in various formats, some of which are
catered to particular religious or philosophical viewpoints. The
following are some of the essential medical topics that are
frequently covered in a living:

- A declaration of personal philosophy or religious values
  to inform medical choices.
- Whether you want artificial respiration and
  cardiopulmonary resuscitation in the case of a
  cardiopulmonary arrest (i.e., whether you want a DNR
  order in place).
- If you cannot eat or drink, whether you want intravenous
  hydration or a feeding tube.
- Your preference about the use of artificial life support in
  the event of a coma or persistent vegetative state.
- Your desire to take part in research studies.
- Whether you consent to an autopsy and donate your
  organs or tissues.

Everyone should ideally have advance directives in place well in
advance of when they are required. Without a living will, an
appointed proxy might make choices against the incapacitated
person's wishes. A living will be interpreted by the next of kin
without a designated proxy, who may or may not decide to follow
its instructions. Without advance directives, the patient's next of
kin will make medical decisions. They must base on the patient's

prior utterances or any known true intentions, values, or religious and philosophical convictions.

Everyone should be aware that intense feelings, familial tensions, and unpredictable circumstances may impact a person's decision-making during a crisis or near the end of their life. Advance directives help everyone navigate challenging situations, but they must also be paired with direct, honest communication between the patient's family and medical team. They must always include a request for the incapacitated person's preferences. However, even if you are caring for someone already experiencing the early stages of an NCD, you can still make advance directives and distribute them to the relevant family members. Discuss with others who would be engaged in medical decision-making if the person is already too impaired to draft the paperwork. Try to agree on what the person would want (or not want) to be done.

A DIRECTORY FOR JURISDICTION

As a conclusion to the preceding section, all caregivers must ensure that the following legal matters are addressed before or during the earliest phases of an NCD:

1. Advance directives should contain a living will, a durable power of attorney for health care decisions, and a chosen health care proxy. Make several copies of these records, and upon admittance, make sure to give copies to your primary care physician, members of your immediate family, and hospitals or long-term care facilities.

2. Financial and estate planning: If the person is already experiencing the beginning stages of an NCD, they should write a will and think about inserting a statement of testamentary ability (perhaps with a videotape). To make it simpler for the agent to act as a surrogate for managing financial assets, prepare a DPOA, and think about opening a joint bank account with the agent. You can select a representative payee, if necessary, to handle government

benefits, or you can arrange for the direct deposit of pensions and other sources of income to that account. Select a reputable attorney as the agent and restrict the obligations outlined in the DPOA agreement if someone is worried about being taken advantage of by relatives or friends or if there will likely be disagreement among children or siblings. If the testator mistrusts a family member who will likely be involved in making decisions, they should expressly limit that person's involvement in the will or living will.

3. Personal values and philosophy: In addition to the very technical and detailed provisions in the document, the will, living will, or separate ethical will can be drafted with a narrative that conveys the person's ideas or philosophy. Following religious legislation, numerous religious organizations have also written particular statements. Close family or friends can be informed in advance, so there is no misunderstanding regarding the individual's genuine preferences.

Final Words

Caring for an individual in the family with dementia is not only challenging but can also be extremely stressful. The situation can even cause depression for those involved in providing care, especially when support is provided at home. Indeed, without a proper guide on what to do, especially in the last stages, things can get extremely confusing and scary.

However, with the knowledge of what one should expect at such stages, things can be made simple through proper planning at every stage. The most important thing to note is that dementia is not a disease with a cure. Instead, it is a term that describes a couple of underlying terminal diseases that are often difficult to treat or manage.

Helping patients with dementia is one of the greatest things a person can do for them when their life changes completely. As discussed in this book, a time comes when they are unable to move their bodies, swallow, sit, or sleep comfortably alone. Being there to help them in such circumstances is an absolute blessing for them, and it can be for you. However, handling their situation without knowing exactly what should be done at each stage can be a challenge. Things can only be easy when you know what to do as a caregiver. Remember that decision-making and communication often become challenging for such patients.

This book was intended to help people who have patients at home suffering from dementia. The most important areas, as shown in this book include symptoms, and, most importantly, what to do as the patient enters the very last stage of dementia and despair begins to set in.

As we come to the end of this book, I hope it has helped you understand all aspects of dementia and has better prepared you to take care of a family member or loved one. The best way to grasp the information in this book is to read again and again or simply refer to it when the need arises.

Thank you for taking the time to educate yourself on this topic further, and I wish you and your family my heartfelt condolences as you embark on this difficult journey of caring for a loved one. If this book has been helpful to you, please share it with others who may be in the same situation with a loved one, or leave a positive review. Again–thank you!

Bibliography

Alzheimer's Association. 2018 Alzheimer's Disease Facts and Figures. Alzheimer's Dementia 2018; 14(3):367-429

Brackey, Jolene. *Creating Moments of Joy Along the Alzheimer's Journey: A Guide for Families and Caregivers*, 5th edition Purdue University Press, 2016.

Branger, C., Burton, R., O'Connell, M. E., Stewart, N., & Morgan, D. (2016). *Coping with cognitive impairment and dementia: Rural caregivers' perspectives.* Dementia, 15(4), 814-831.

Brooker, D. (2003). What is person-centered care in dementia?. Reviews in clinical gerontology, 13(3), 215-222.

Engdahl, S. (2013). Dementia. Greenhaven Publishing LLC.

Goodreads. (1970, January 1). *Dementia caregiver guide by TEEPA Snow*. Goodreads. Retrieved June 29, 2022, from https://www.goodreads.com/book/show/40663808-dementia-caregiver-guide

Kovach, C.R. (1997). Late-Stage Dementia: A Basic Guide. Taylor & Francis.

Mitchell, Wendy, and Anna Wharton. *Somebody I Used to Know: A Memoir*. Ballantine Books, an Imprint of Random House, 2018.

Stephen Garrard Post. 2000. *The Moral Challenge of Alzheimer's Disease: Ethical Issues from Diagnosis to Dying*. Baltimore: Johns Hopkins University Press.

Passages in Caregiving: Turning Chaos into Confidence, by Gail Sheehy (William Morrow, 2010).

Paula Spencer Scott. 2014. *Surviving Alzheimer's: Practical Tips and Soul-Saving Wisdom for Caregivers*. Eva Birch Media.